READ THIS BOOK IF...

- You or a loved one is unwell – physically emotionally or mentally.
- You have no idea whether or not God heals today.
- You're absolutely convinced divine healing is not for today.
- You believe in divine healing but are having trouble receiving it.
- You believe illness is ultimately the devil's fault.
- You believe illness is from God, or that He allows it.
- You have no theological education whatsoever.
- You're a pastor, priest, minister, missionary, or attended seminary/Bible college.
- You know there must be more to God than what you've experienced so far.
- You pray for people and want to see them healed, but lack confidence or have not seen successful outcomes yet.
- You love to hear testimonies of healing.
- You want to avoid illness.
- You want answers as to why your loved one died.
- You hear contradictions in what you're taught at church.
- You have seen contradictions and hypocrisy in the church, so are no longer interested in God. And yet...something is missing in your life, including health.

MORE BY KEMALA TRIBE

The Head-Smacker Series
Disarming Deadly Doctrines – Stop Sickness in its Tracks with Head-Smacking Revelations of God's Will
Deceptive Doctrines (working title - upcoming)
Doctrines of Demons (working title - upcoming)

Other Non-Fiction in Progress
Everyday God
(working title – collection of first-hand signs and wonders)

Fiction
"Summer Breeze"
Awarded publication in
"Southern Writers Best Short Fiction 2015"

"Daddy Knows"
Published in Chicken Soup for the Soul's
"Dreams and the Unexplainable"

BONUS CONTENT
@ kemalatribe.ca

To download gifts such as
   Printable confession cards
   List of healing scriptures
   Book - Healing Action Plan
   Books by guest authors
   Inspiring short stories
   And more (will vary, visit often),
go to kemalatribe.ca and join my mailing list. You will also receive devotionals chock full of head-smacking revelations! I promise I won't clog your inbox -- only one or two per month.

DISARMING DEADLY DOCTRINES

Stop Sickness in its Tracks with
Head-Smacking Revelations of God's Will

Book One in the Head-Smacker Series by
KEMALA B. TRIBE

Copyright © 2020 by Kemala Tribe

All rights reserved. No part of this publication may be reproduced, distributed or transmitted in any form or by any means, including photocopying, recording, or other electronic or mechanical methods without the prior written permission of the publisher, except in the case of brief quotations in reviews and certain other non-commercial uses permitted by copyright law.

Printed in USA

First Printing, 2020

ISBN 978-1-7771885-0-4 print
ISBN 978-1-7771885-1-1 eBook
ISBN 978-1-7771885-2-8 audio

www.kemalatribe.ca

WingShadow Publishing
BC, CANADA

Legally required disclaimer: *The content of this book is for informational purposes only and is not intended to diagnose, treat, cure, or prevent any condition or disease. You understand that this book is not intended as a substitute for consultation with a licensed practitioner. Please consult with your own physician or healthcare specialist regarding the suggestions and recommendations made in this book. The use of this book implies your acceptance of this disclaimer.*

For Bible Translation copyright information and abbreviations, please see back matter.

To my Kevin —

*How I wish we could have
written this book together.
And yet you've been with me in every word.*

Thank you, Father, for making your will so clear...

Every word you give me is a miracle word—
how could I help but obey?
Break open your words, let the light shine out,
let ordinary people see the meaning.
Psalm 119:129,130 - The Message

TABLE OF CONTENTS

Read This Book If... i
More By Kemala Tribe ii
Foreword xi
A Note From The Author xiii
Pointers For Using This Book xv
Introduction xvii

PART ONE
Your Health Is Vital In God's Plan 1

Chapter 1 Is God's Will For You Revealed? 3
               Jesus Came To Execute God's Will 7
Chapter 2 What You Don't Know About Sovereignty Can Kill You 11
Chapter 3 Is There More To Redemption? 15
               Two Things You Must Be Assured Of 15
               Our Salvation 20
               Isaiah Vs The Apostles On Healing 24
               But Wait, There's More 26

PART TWO
Remember The Great Things He Has Done 29

Chapter 4 As You Believe, So Be It 31
Chapter 5 Real-Life Examples 35
               Cured Of The Incurable 35
               Kevin's Leg – Healed 36
               Kevin's Leg – Restored 38
               Trial By Fire – Mom's Arm 39
               The Easiest Thing To Pray For 40
               Stand Your Ground 40

PART THREE
God's Word Is True 43

Chapter 6 Why Don't We Take God's Word At Face Value? 45
        You're Being Sabotaged! 48

Chapter 7 Settling God's Word 55
        Seeing Isn't Always Believing 58
        The Proof Is Relationship 60

Chapter 8 Wash Your Brain 65
        Scripture As Medicine 68
        The Father's Desire 69

PART FOUR
Deadly Doctrines: Man's Wisdom, The Enemy's Lies 73

Chapter 9 Holding On To Human Traditions 75
        9 Head-Smackers that Prove God Wants You Healed 80

Chapter 10 Healing Is Not For Today 87
        Healing Manifests In Heaven 87
        But That Was Jesus 90
        Miracles Died With The Apostles 92

Chapter 11 Unworthiness 103
        I'm Not Worthy 103
        I Must Have Done Something Wrong 105
        My Sin Blocks The Blessings 106
        He's Teaching Me A Lesson (Disciplining Me In Love) 110

Chapter 12 God Is Sovereign 115
        God Gets The Glory For My Suffering 115
        Suffering For Jesus 116
        Suffering As Job Did 118
        He's Calling Me Home 120
        God Is Saving Her From What's Ahead 123
        God Makes Us Ill For Unknown Reasons 125

    God Hurts Us So He Can Show Off Later 126
    Satan Has No Power Over My Body 128
Chapter 13 He's Able But Is He Willing? 131
    Questioning God's Intent Toward You................................... 131
    If God Wants Me Healed, He'll Heal Me 132
    Paul's Thorn 135
    God Didn't Heal Timothy 137
    I Brought This On Myself... 140
    It Isn't Always His Will To Heal.. 142
Chapter 14 He's Willing But Is He Able? 145
    It Runs In The Family 145
    Jesus Couldn't Heal In Nazareth... 148
    He Can Heal Some Things, But Not Your Thing.................. 150
    If I Only Had Enough Faith.. 151
Chapter 15 Praying "...If It Be Thy Will" 157

PART FIVE
Your Transformed Mind In Action 159
Chapter 16 Hope Again 161
    Go On The Offensive 162
    Defensive Measures 163
    Tactical Maneuvers... 164
Chapter 17 The Vision 167

Acknowledgements 175
Bible Translations And Copyrights 177

FOREWORD

You don't often find someone willing to take the time to search out the scriptures for answers to what you've often had questions about. Kemala Tribe has taken the time to do this in "Disarming Deadly Doctrines -- Stop Sickness in its Tracks with Head-Smacking Revelations of God's Will." These writings put the practice of everyday, unfailing faith within the believer's grasp.

This book is faith-building, inspiring, informative, and most of all it reaches the highest standard of truth. Kemala has written a great book for establishing the understanding and use of scripture, and to inform the practical use of applicable understanding. No matter at what level of faith you may find yourself, reading Disarming Deadly Doctrines will answer many questions you may have concerning healing in the Bible. More than that, it will reveal the patterns by which you can open the understanding of the scriptures for yourself. Kemala will demonstrate through her personal interaction with these principles how to make the scriptures come alive and work on your behalf. She shares personal healings and testimonies of other's miracles after employing these patterns. The insights she shares in this book can truly lead to a higher level of fleshing out, in the natural, God's intentions for you in the Spiritual.

On a personal note, I pastored Kemala and her husband Kevin many years ago. They were a beautiful couple with great plans ahead to serve God. As I watched them grow spiritually, I saw many great things in store for them prophetically. But Kevin, a great Kingdom warrior, unexpectedly went on to meet his heavenly reward. It's incredible to watch how Kemala has beautifully picked up the pieces to fulfill her Kingdom call. She has so much experience to share. I wouldn't miss reading a book by this woman of faith.

Pastor Beth Bonner Th.M.

A NOTE FROM THE AUTHOR

Just a day or two into what I thought was going to be a three-page essay, I knew I had a book on my hands and in my heart. For every statement I typed, I heard in my mind a countering question. For every question I answered, I heard a skeptic's, "But..." So I kept writing. I wanted to settle every "but." I told the Lord that I wouldn't send this book to print until every point He wanted me to make had been addressed. He kept revealing more and more until I thought I'd never finish!

I certainly do not know everything there is to know about divine healing, but I have faith that everything God wants me to share with you at this time is within these pages. Every time I open this book, I learn something new — and I WROTE it! So don't read this book only once.

This endeavor has substantially increased my Bible reading and engendered a renewed passion for scripture. One word from God, often by a tiny Holy Spirit tweak in perspective, is all it takes to change your life. So strap in, folks, because this read is going to be an adventurous treasure hunt! I'm very grateful to the Lord for placing this task before me and leading me through it. It has been as much a blessing to me as I hope it will be to you.

Your Sister in Christ,

Kemala

...And for me, that utterance may be given to me, that I may open my mouth boldly to make known the mystery of the gospel - Ephesians 6:19 NKJV

POINTERS FOR USING THIS BOOK

First things first — pray. Open your heart; tell the Holy Spirit you long to renew your mind to His truth. Tell Him you want everything He has for you — that you're willing, as long as it comes from God, to receive something you've never heard before.

For this series of books, I have broadened the definition of *doctrine* to simply this: *a belief or teaching common among Christians today*. Some of these doctrines are found in certain groups, i.e., charismatics, or particular denominations. Others are prevalent throughout the church. Some may not be taught by any church, yet are assumed to be valid by many individuals due to personal experience and lack of correct teaching in that area.

Don't do like I used to do — skip the scriptures and read just the author's writing. When the light bulbs flash on in your mind, WOW — you'll never look at scripture as boring again! They will change your life; they will change your body. In fact, they literally have life in them.

If you see a word in bold or capital letters within a passage of scripture, I'm calling your attention to something important. I may also toss in a little something extra in parentheses. I am fully aware that *satan* is a proper noun, but to my editor's chagrin, I stubbornly refuse to capitalize it. And out of respect, I always capitalize *Bible*.

A very detailed table of contents has been provided so that after your first reading, this book can be used as a reference. For this purpose, each section needs to stand on its own, so you'll find some repetition of points and of scriptures.

Fair warning: the truths I am putting forward may be a paradigm shift for you, and the Bible warns that the true gospel is offensive to many. So take every point to the Lord with the pursuit of His truth in your heart. See what He says about it. And if my style feels too aggressive to you, please consider that this boldness may be exactly what is required for another person to catch what God has for him. My aim is only and always to bless you — to share what has been revealed to me — in obedience to God.

At any point during your reading, when you feel a revelation hit your soul, receive your healing! Don't wait for the end of the book or the next church service, just receive. Continue reading to garner all that's in here for you, but don't wait a second longer than necessary to get healthy — physically, mentally, emotionally and spiritually. Be whole (Shalom).

INTRODUCTION

Why did Jesus heal them all in His day, but leave you to struggle with illness in the here and now? Why is it we see an all-powerful God in the Bible Who rescued His people every other chapter, yet nothing ever seems to change in YOUR life? Is pain going to plague you the rest of your days? Is the abundant life unachievable?

With the results most of us see in our day-to-day, it's no wonder we think of God as far away, uninterested in what we're dealing with. It can feel like He leaves us to slog through the muck of this world until we die and finally see His goodness in heaven. It's an exhausting life! Unless…

Might there be more to this whole Christianity thing than we hear about most Sunday mornings? Is there something we're missing — something even our church leadership may be missing? Within these pages, you'll find answers that have been right there in God's Word all along, and He's going to reveal them to you today.

You've probably heard all your life that God helps those who help themselves, that we have to have a certain amount of faith to receive healing, or that healing isn't for today. You were likely taught that it isn't always God's will to heal, proven by Paul's thorn and Timothy's frequent infirmities. I was raised on all the same beliefs, taught by well-intentioned theologians.

From now on, though, take God's word for it, not your teachers'! Had I known ten years ago what I know now, I would not have buried my husband. You don't have to go through what we went through. Determination to find out what we had missed, that lack of knowledge that had led to what I knew was not God's best for us, has culminated in this book you're holding.

From Jan Mason, editor of this book

It all started when Kemala came to visit us. My husband, Steve, was having recurring afib (heart rate in the 180-190 range) even though he'd had an ablation just a few weeks before. Kemala told me about the book she was writing on believing God regarding healing, and we talked about healing Steve. I knew about her personal healings, but being a cradle Catholic, I had never considered that I might facilitate a healing.

Steve weakened to the point that he couldn't walk from the bed to the sofa without resting. After his second trip to the hospital, it was time to make a decision, and I decided to put what I had learned from Kemala to use. Steve was placed in Cardiac Observation, where he had been twice before. When he hadn't gotten out of bed for over a day, and although he was a man with a large appetite, hadn't eaten anything in two days, his doctor became concerned that he may have suffered some heart damage during the ablation. That night, the technologists were busy performing tests to diagnose the extent of damage his doctor thought he must have. That's when I got to work, praying in my own words what Kemala had explained. I had never spoken to God so boldly before, but I was desperate for Steve to get well. I sat in his hospital room and prayed over him while he slept, believing and expecting God to heal him.

The next morning at 5:00, he woke up, got out of bed, turned the lights on, and walked down the hall to the bathroom. When he came back into the room, I noticed that his color was normal again, and he didn't look tired. He said he was hungry and wondered if he could get some breakfast.

The nurse got him breakfast, and we waited for his doctor to come in on his morning rounds. He told us that he was happy to say that all of the tests came back showing no visible heart damage. He seemed somewhat surprised. So I told him I believed Steve had been healed.

I asked God to give me a sign that he was indeed healed. A small voice in my head kept repeating, "Steve is healed." Anytime I got quiet that day and for many days to come, I heard that voice say, "Steve is healed."

A year later, he is still afib free. The doctor confirmed it – Steve is healed!

Whether it's your own condition or that of a loved one, whether it's migraines or depression, infertility or kidney stones, stage 5 cancer or a sprained ankle, after reading this book, you'll see God and His intentions toward you from a fresh and joyous perspective. Exciting revelations will usher you into a healthy new lease on life. With one who's been right where you are today, dive headfirst into the living water of the revelation of LIFE as God intended it to be for us here on earth. You'll find that abundant life Jesus said He came to give us.

DISARMING DEADLY DOCTRINES

PART ONE
Your Health is Vital in God's Plan

Dear friend, I am praying that everything prosper with you and that you be in good health, as I know you are prospering spiritually. - 3 John 1:2 CJB

"With a long life I will satisfy him and let him see My salvation." - Psalm 91:16 NASB

Good people suffer many troubles, but the LORD saves them from them all; - Psalm 34:19 GNT

"For I know the plans I have for you" — this is the LORD's declaration — "plans for your well-being, not for disaster, to give you a future and a hope."
- Jeremiah 29:11 CSB

CHAPTER ONE
Is God's Will For You Revealed?

Head-smackers — that's what I've found, time and time again, in research for this book. It's those moments when you say, "How have I never seen that? Was that there all along? How could I have missed that?" Or just plain, "Duh." One hundred percent of those moments have either been while reading scriptures or meditating on them. For a long time, I wasn't much of a Bible reader, sporadic at best. But now I know — it's a living, breathing, blessing encyclopedia! Everything we need is in there, and it's all good.

God's Word Is God's Will

For example, where would you look to find out what God has promised you? If you want to know what all Christians are called to do in this life, where would you find that information? What is God's will regarding tithing, sex, drinking, business practices, marriage, paying taxes? Your go-to source of information, applying to us all as Christians is, of course, the Bible, and every word of it is for our benefit. It's all good because God is good. Most Christians agree, whether our actions confirm it or not, that the Bible is inspired — the unerring, God-breathed word of our almighty, omnipotent, omniscient, omnipresent God. It's His Word you need to consult for answers in every area of life, because God's Word is God's Will.

That simple but profound statement changed my world. It made Scripture come to life again after a spiritual drought. It renewed my zeal for the Word and showed me two things that should have been obvious from the beginning:

- You can only know God's will if you know God's word.
- You must believe that God said what He meant and meant what He said.

The scriptures on the Part One title page may sound untrue to you. Perhaps you believe you've put them to the test in your life and were disappointed. But you must always be careful to read scripture in context and to examine any promise of God to see if it has conditions or instructions for making it work in your life.

The key, though, is this: you have to truly believe the word. And, you **must** mix it with faith.

> For we have heard the Good News, just as they did. They
> heard the message, but it did them no good, because when
> they heard it, they did not accept it with faith.
> - Hebrews 4:2 GNT

God has zero intention of tricking you. His word is absolutely true. So be careful that you are not making assumptions and then blaming God for the unavoidable disappointment they caused.

> So is My word that goeth out of My mouth, it turns not
> back unto Me empty, But hath done that which I desired,
> And **prosperously effected** that for which I sent it.
> - Isaiah 55:11 YLT

> Then the LORD said to me, "Right. I am watching to make
> sure that my words come true." - Jeremiah 1:12 GW

Amazing scriptures from an amazing God. Knowing He has to cause them to come to pass, God chose His words very carefully. Right now is the time to decide that everything God says in His Word is truth, and it is truth regardless of the circumstance staring back at you, regardless of what other people say it means. Until you do that, you cannot see it ***prosperously affect*** any area of your life, including health.

> ...Let God be found veracious and every man a liar, even as
> it stands written, To the end that you may be acknowledged
> in your words, and may come out victor when brought to
> trial. - Romans 3:4 WET

Agreeing with God, even to the point that you have to consider every human a liar, will prove you right in the end.

> Jesus did not heal the sick in order to coax them to be
> Christians. He healed because it was His nature to heal.
> - John G. Lake

First and foremost, you must get to know His nature and character. That is Job #1 as Christians. The Bible is our primary resource for this pursuit. In reading the Bible, when you come to a word or phrase that's unfamiliar, define the Bible by the Bible. This means look up other places where that original word is used in the scriptures in order to help you understand the Biblical meaning of the word. Look back to the original ancient Hebrew or Greek from which the Bible was translated to glean the true meaning as even our English has changed a lot over the centuries. God has provided tools (concordances, lexicons, dictionaries, etc.) so that you can search out the mysteries and understand Him correctly, and now they're available online for free.

When you get saved, you ask the Holy Spirit to dwell in you, and going forward from that moment, you should ask Him to help you understand the scriptures as you read them. It's part of developing your personal relationship with God, which is His heart's desire. Then, when you feel you've heard from Him in a personal way, you can authenticate that rhema word by checking it against scripture. This is an effective strategy when you're learning to recognize His voice.

I'm going to inject a cautionary statement here. If you research online, know that there is a lot of teaching that does not line up with the scriptures. It will sound good; it may come from a reputable source. But sometimes even trusted names in the Body are believing the lies they were taught. Remember, ask the Holy Spirit to teach you, and know that if it isn't speaking life to your soul, it isn't God.

But why is knowing His will crucial to you at this moment in time? Because without the knowledge of God's will for you, your faith cannot operate! If you're not **confident** that what you're praying for is God's will, your prayers will be faithless and ineffective. It is the prayer of faith that saves the sick,

Step #1 to Effective Use of Scripture: Start Believing It

according to James 5. Furthermore, you must not only know that the thing you desire is God's will in a general sense, you must know in your heart that it is His will for YOU. Otherwise, doubt creeps in and spoils everything. By the time you've finished this book, you'll put scripture, which is living and is God's "power unto salvation" (Romans 1:16), to work for you to bring about God's good plan for your life.

Can we agree that God wants His plan for your life to come to fruition? I'd say that's a no-brainer. If He planned it, it's obviously what He wants. Can we agree that God's plan for your life is His best for you? It's two ways of saying the same thing. Now, can we agree that His scriptures are His way of pointing you down the right path toward His best for you? So far, we're probably on the same page. He says we are to be doers of the Word, not just hearers (James 2:14-24, 26). So by doing the Word, you're moving along His path toward His best plan for you, right?

But, you have to gain understanding of what the Word means in order to progress. Come on now, you know you do it, too. You've read scriptures over and over and not really granted that the words mean what they say. I know I've done it — still do sometimes. The word sounds good, but you aren't really digesting it and applying it in your life. Or you get to a familiar passage and skim over it mentally, because you think you know what it means.

> My son, pay attention to my words; incline your ear to my sayings. Do not lose sight of them; keep them within your heart. For they are life to those who find them, and health to the whole BODY. - Proverbs 4:20-22 CSB

Slow down, read each word, and think about what God is saying. Be one of those *who find them* so you will understand what God has made available to you as a believer. You must read the Word and then perceive its meaning with the Holy Spirit's help — that is *finding* it. That's when you can renew your mind with it and apply it in your own personal, everyday life. When you actually perceive it, it will blow you away. God is too good to be true, yet He is. And note that God says, "My son..." in the scripture above. He's addressing those already in the Kingdom, already His children and heirs. At the time, those were the Jews, but now that includes us grafted-in Christians.

Being a Christian, if you are, attending church for decades, even serving as an elder, deacon or pastor, doesn't mean you have an accurate picture in your mind of God, of His nature and character. If in your mind, God isn't exactly like the Jesus portrayed in the New Testament, then you don't have an accurate view of God.

> The Son is the image of the invisible God, the firstborn over all creation. - Colossians 1:15 BSB

> Jesus saith unto him, Have I been so long time with you, and yet hast thou not known me, Philip? he that hath seen me hath seen the Father; and how sayest thou then, Shew us the Father? - John 14:9 KJV

God Speaks LIFE and Only Life Over You

Scripture testifies that Jesus is the exact image of the Father and of His nature. If you don't fully comprehend that, you will not perceive the scriptures the way He intends. You can carry on conversations with the Father daily but be filtering everything He says through your own understanding and miss some of His goodness. The Word and knowing His character are essential to discovering His will for your life.

Incline your ear to His Word, not just to your preacher or teacher. I'm not down on pastors or teachers. I know their intentions are good. But sometimes, in teaching what they've been taught, they're propagating error. If the voice you're listening to is not speaking life to you the way Jesus spoke (boundless hope, effective faith, overwhelming love, absolute promises), then the words are not inspired by God. God says His Word brings life, and His gospel is the power unto salvation. That, in a nutshell, is His will for you revealed. Remember that Jesus IS the Word, the Word made flesh, the daily Bread of Life, and He came to execute our Father's will on this earth. He is our example, and He reveals God's will. What He did on earth is what we're supposed to receive and do because the Father is unchangeable.

Jesus Came to Execute God's Will

Hopefully we all have it firmly established in our hearts that Jesus is:
- One third of the triune Godhead,
- The only begotten son of God,
- Completely man and completely God,
- God's Word transformed into a flesh and blood man,
- The only perfect, sinless man to ever walk this earth,
- The propitiation (atoning sacrifice) for our sins.

> The Son radiates God's own glory and expresses the very character of God, and he sustains everything by the mighty power of his command. When he had cleansed us from our sins, he sat down in the place of honor at the right hand of the majestic God in heaven. - Hebrews 1:3 NLT

The AMPC says it this way: ...the sole expression of the glory of God ...the out-raying of the divine...the perfect imprint and very image of (God's) nature... That explains so eloquently that when you look at Jesus' life and ministry, you see the Father's will being accomplished and His character illuminated for all to see — for you to see.

> "For I came down from heaven, not to do mine own will, but the will of him that sent me." - John 6:38 KJV

> "Then I said, 'Behold, I have come — In the volume of the book it is written of Me — To do Your will, O God.'"
> - Hebrews 10:7,9 NKJV

> For I have never spoken on My own initiative or authority; but the Father Himself who sent Me has given Me a commandment regarding what to say and what to speak.
> - John 12:49 AMP

There can be no doubt — whatever you saw Jesus do, it was the will of the Father.

> When evening had come, they brought to Him many who were demon-possessed. And He cast out the spirits with a word, and healed all who were sick, that it might be fulfilled which was spoken by Isaiah the prophet, saying: "He Himself took our infirmities and bore our sicknesses."
> - Matthew 8:16,17 NKJV

When Jesus was here, it didn't matter what disease anyone had. It didn't matter if it was contagious. It didn't matter if it was a congenital birth defect or an acquired illness. It didn't matter if it was viral, fungal, parasitical or bacterial or an allergic reaction. It didn't matter if it was life-threatening or just a nuisance. It didn't matter how many generations that condition had been plaguing the family.

It didn't matter who the person was and whether or not they came from a *good* family. It didn't matter their looks, their lifestyle or their *level* of sin. He never said, "Talk to me about healing after you've cleaned up your life," or "Move out of that man's tent, then we'll talk about healing." He never said, "Go and sin no more for forty days, and then I'll heal you." He didn't say, "Believe in Me, so when you get to heaven you'll be healed."

Here's another thing He never said — "Confess your sins, and I'll heal you." (see note at chapter end).

That's a shocker! Jesus healed multitudes — too many to count — so it's a pretty fair bet that those He healed included a murderer or two, rapists and lots of adulterers. We know the Jews at that time hated Samaritans, so there were racists. There certainly would have been gossips, and gossip is a big deal to God. There had to have been liars and cheats and hypocrites. There were those who coveted their neighbors' spouses and possessions. And since there are no new sins today, what about women who'd aborted their babies? Yes, there were those, too, by whatever means they used back then. And there would have been the abortionists, too.

Jesus healed them all. Whatever you saw Jesus do for others is God's will for you, too.

Note: James linked healing and confession, but confession to one another — a totally different subject. The context of James 5 is of personal relationships — confess your faults one to another so that you can forgive each other and work in unity as the body of Christ.

CHAPTER 2
What You Don't Know About Sovereignty Can Kill You

Do you believe that God is sovereign? That He can do anything at any time and nobody can interfere with Him? That everything that happens, happens because it is His will? That we have no control over what that might be, nor could we stop it if we wanted to? This is the belief of many Christians, but is it an accurate portrayal of what Almighty God has put in motion?

In Genesis 1:28, God says He made us and gave us dominion over all the earth and every living thing that moves on it. I looked up the definition of *dominion,* and I was blown away. It's so much more robust than I knew.

> Dominion: supremacy, ascendancy, dominance, domination, superiority, predominance, preeminence, primacy, hegemony, authority, mastery, control, command, direction, power, sway, rule, government, jurisdiction, lordship, **sovereignty**, overlordship, leadership, influence; the upper hand, the whip hand, the edge, advantage, hold, grasp. (*googledictionary.com*)

Staggering, isn't it? And there's that word *sovereignty* again. God, Who is sovereign, gave YOU His sovereignty here on the earth He prepared for you. He just handed it over! So you have dominion, or sovereignty, on earth. Huh.

There's no doubt that God's ultimate plan — as many people saved as possible, Jesus' return, the millennial reign, heaven on earth, eternity in your place of choice (I choose mansions, how about you?) — will come to pass. The scriptures tell us that nothing can stop the plans of God.

So how do those two facts — God's sovereignty and yours — coexist? It's simple. God restrained His own dominion here, because the earth was His gift to us. A gift has no strings attached. That's how Adam could lose the keys (that authority) to satan when he and Eve sinned. If God had retained ultimate authority, the devil could not have appropriated that authority from Adam and Eve. It wouldn't have been theirs to lose. So God came as a man under the law to overturn the rule of the enemy and take back everything Adam had lost.

Believe, Speak, Expect — Use Your Dominion

We're in charge again! Well, to be clear, dominion has been restored to those of us who are in Christ. In the New Testament, God tells YOU, to deal with the devil. "Resist the devil and he will flee from you" (James 4:7). Notice he flees from YOU. But you can enlist God's help through prayer, and He will fight your battles. He calls you His hands and feet in this world. He calls you to give toward good works and sow seed in fertile ground, and He empowers you through the Holy Spirit to do good works. He is very involved in the earth, but we have dominion here. That's why you can declare a thing, and it will be so. Your words are creative because you are made in His image, and you have been given the authority to do so as His child. Check this out - it's amazing:

> Ye are blessed of the Lord which made heaven and earth. The heaven, even the heavens, are the Lord's: **but the earth hath he given to the children of men**.
> - Psalm 115:15,16 KJV

Wow! Is this a change of perspective for you? I know it is for a lot of people, but it's right there in the Bible:

> And God blessed them, and God said unto them, Be fruitful, and multiply, and replenish the earth, and subdue it: and have dominion over the fish of the sea, and over the fowl of the air, and over every living thing that moveth upon the earth. - Genesis 1:28 KJV

Please note there were no other people at that time. We are not given dominion over people. That is called despotism.

> Since by the one man's trespass, death reigned through that one man, how much more will those who receive the overflow of grace and the gift of righteousness reign in life through the one man, Jesus Christ. - Romans 5:17 CSB

> I tell you the truth, whatever you forbid on earth will be forbidden in heaven, and whatever you permit on earth will be permitted in heaven. -Matthew 18:18 NLT

> Behold, I give you the authority... over all the power of the enemy, and nothing shall hurt you. - Luke 10:19 ESV

You've Got the Power!

How does this dominion affect you in your daily life? To be honest, it puts the onus on you. It makes you personally responsible for your circumstances. You can't blame God for how your life is going if you have dominion on earth. However, God wouldn't give you this responsibility without the power to accomplish whatever needs to be done. That just wouldn't be good management. He also promises to be with you and gives you The Helper. We are not God. We need the guidance of our Father and our Big Brother. And without the help of the Holy Spirit, we can accomplish nothing.

Have you ever wondered about the prophets in the Old Testament, how it was possible for them to do miracles? Have you asked yourself why the Bible never says that God TOLD Elijah to call down fire? God told Moses to stretch out His arm, but there seem to be just as many instances of the prophets taking the initiative on their own and thinking up ways to show God mighty. There are two reasons for that: 1) they knew God's will (what He wanted to accomplish), and 2) they knew God had given them authority with their position — so He would back them up with power. It's time we, meaning you and me, started using the authority Jesus gave us, and the power living inside us, the Holy Spirit.

We're going to touch on how to effect change and enforce God's will in Part Five. For now, just keep in mind as you read, that you have been deputized by Jesus. You are authorized to enforce the will of our Heavenly Father in this world, including in your own life and circumstances. It's the same deputization (dominion) Adam received. Feeling the power?

CHAPTER 3
Is There More to Redemption?

When the American Medical Association was founded in 1847, the serpent on the staff was chosen as their logo. Why? Thousands of years earlier, in the wilderness, the Israelites suffered the attack of venomous snakes. But God made a way out for them — in Numbers 21:8-9, God instructed Moses to make a bronze serpent and lift it high on a pole. Bronze represents judgement, and the serpent (the enemy) being lifted on the staff was a picture of the judgement of satan when Jesus would be lifted up on the cross. All anyone bitten by the poisonous snakes had to do was look up at the bronze serpent, in effect observing Jesus' work on the cross to come, and they were healed. That is how powerful Jesus' finished work is. That alone — the serpent on the cross healing the Israelites — is proof that healing is in the atonement.

God always exhorted the Israelites to *choose life* and declared Himself the God that heals, even under the Old Covenant. Now we're under the New Covenant, the covenant that declares the real cross has judged the real enemy and taken away any authority he used to have. Jesus paid a dear price to give you the New Covenant in His blood. Don't waste it.

Two Things You Must be Assured Of

The dearth of understanding in the church on these two subjects – God's love for you and the source of sickness and disease – is shocking, and explains why the church as a whole is sick and lacking. You will never hear me say that our lives as Christians should be soft and comfortable. No, if we're doing Christianity right, we should be embattled every day, to some degree, even if we are only laboring to remain in His rest. But the nature of God is to give, and it is His great delight to pour out His grace and blessing on you — from freedom to wisdom, from divine appointments to new friendships, from health to houses, from peace to profits. He wants all good things for you, even to the point of preparing you spiritually to be able to be good stewards of what He wants to bless you with.

We all know the scripture, "my people are destroyed for lack of knowledge" (Hosea 4-6 KJV), but do you realize it is literally true? Christians are literally dying because they have no idea that God wants them healed more than they themselves want to be healed. A deeper understanding of the following two subjects will help Christians and non-Christians alike to grasp this.

1. God's Love for You

As humans we simply don't have the same capacity for love that God has, so we have trouble comprehending how great that love is. He IS love. Our triune God loves you more than your parents love you, more than your spouse loves you, and more than you love your children — more than you love yourself.

Who besides Jesus would endure torture and death for you? You have God's undivided attention 24/7. He thinks about you constantly. He wants to deepen His relationship with you, to communicate with you all day, every day. He wants to bless your every endeavor. He wants to increase your ability and capacity to receive from Him. You are the apple of His eye, His favorite. He adores you. He knows everything about you, and loves you anyway. He planned you even before the foundations of the earth. Nothing you do will make Him love you less. Nothing you do will make Him love you more because His love for you is already complete and everlasting. You cannot escape it. It is irrefutable and overwhelming. He is so excited about you and your future together!

If you are saved, He has sent His Spirit of Life to take up residence inside you. He has given you the gift of righteousness, the measure of faith, and made you a new creation. You're a new species that never existed before Jesus — a mortal body enveloping the Spirit of God. He has adopted you into His family and given you the same inheritance as His Son, and He paid a very high price for you. He has given you every good thing, every spiritual gift in heavenly places, even resurrection power inside of you. He has predestined you for success and seated you with Jesus on High. He has proclaimed that nothing can separate you from His love and has sent His angels to camp around you and protect you. He has given you His Name. He has anointed you, set you apart. He has given you the mind of Christ, a spirit of power, of love, and of a sound mind. He has accepted you in the Beloved. How could anything prevail against you? He helps you. He steps into every weak spot and shows you how to be strong in Him when you allow Him to. You are more than a conqueror — you get to go in after His victory and collect the loot. You are highly favored, greatly blessed, and deeply loved. He defeated death and every evil thing at the cross on your behalf. The whole time He was suffering, He was thinking of you and the impact He was making in your life. There is no love greater than the love He has for you.

2. The Source of Illness and Death

We humans get into trouble from page one in Genesis, and I do not mean Adam & Eve. I'm talking about the church — you and me. If we doubt God in Genesis, we'll doubt Him throughout the Bible. And this doubt stems from our misinterpretation right out of the gate.

We think, and we're taught, that what God said and what God meant are two different things. We wonder why Adam and Eve didn't drop dead at the base of the Tree of the Knowledge of Good and Evil when they ate the forbidden fruit. King James said they would surely die, but they lived! The reason we question what we think of as their survival? We forget that Adam and Eve were created immortal in their human bodies. They were **never** going to die before their disobedience.

> You Now Have God's DNA
> New Father
> New Family
> New Species

But the ancient Hebrew text does not say, "you will surely die." It says, "Dying, you shall die." What does *dying* mean to you? Aging? Sickness? Yes, aging and disease are incipient death, death coming closer and closer every day. Adam and Eve by sin lost their immortality — their physical bodies were no longer eternal. They began to age. They became susceptible to decay and disease. Perfection was destroyed. The Adamic covenant had been breached. This is what we call The Fall. Dying, they eventually died. **God said exactly what He meant. WE misinterpreted it.**

So we made up our own explanations for what we decided God must have meant. Our story about why Adam and Eve didn't die the day they disobeyed? "Well, you see, they died spiritually, not physically. God is spirit, so when He says death, He means spiritual death." That one fallacy has caused generations of Christians to doubt the Word of God. It has also colored our understanding of every scripture containing the word *death*, causing us to spiritualize them. Inevitably, it also caused us to misunderstand the word *life*. We have continued to employ that interpretive process of 1) misunderstand, 2) think up an explanation by man's wisdom, 3) thereby cause another misunderstanding, 4) repeat. We've used it down through the centuries, and we've used it from Genesis to Revelation.

There is a better way: believe the Word first. Listen, folks. From now on, when you come across something in scripture that sounds contradictory, that sounds like God made a mistake, or anything that does not seem to reflect well on God, know that the error is in your understanding or that of the person you're learning from. Further investigation and asking the Holy Spirit for revelation will bring clarity. God is always right.

Now, what's the problem with our thinking that God meant spiritual death for Adam and Eve? For centuries we haven't understood the connection between sin and physical death, and therefore, we have misconstrued God's stance on physical death, sickness, disease and aging.

> Wherefore, as by one man sin entered into the world, and death by sin; - Romans 5:12 KJV

Is there anything else that need be said? Death entered the earth on the back of sin. Had there been no sin, there would be no death. The Greek word translated *death* here is *thanatos* — the death of the body — not spiritual death! In *Strong's Concordance*, it's word #*G2288*:
1. The death of the body
   a. That separation (whether natural or violent) of the soul and the body by which the life on earth is ended
   b. With the implied idea of future misery in hell You can see that the secondary definition 'b' even ties physical death to sin.

To compound the error, spiritual death is not only inaccurate in the case of Adam and Eve, but defining it as separation from God, causes the assumption that when we sin we are separated from God — exactly the time we need to be closest to Him. What was God's response when Adam and Eve sinned? He still visited them, they still carried on a conversation. They were NOT separated from Him. This second fallacy has further distanced us from the Lord Whose greatest desire is to be in intimate relationship with each of us individually. God Himself killed animals to cover Adam and Eve's sin-debt, and then He made clothes for them from the animal skins. Does that sound like separation from God to you?

The sacrificial animals paid by their physical deaths, not spiritual deaths, and continued to be killed as sacrificial payment to cover sin until Jesus came and died physically on the cross to pay for all sin for all time. The animals died physically and Jesus died physically. Why would we ever think that Adam and Eve did not die physically as a result of sin?

> [In fact] under the Law almost everything is purified by means of blood, and without the shedding of blood there is neither release from sin and its guilt nor the remission of the due and merited punishment for sins.
> - Hebrews 9:22 AMPC

So if sin requires a payment of physical death (the shedding of blood), then, of course, physical death entered the earth with sin! They go hand in hand. And where does sin originate? With our enemy, who comes only to **KILL**, steal and destroy.

> You know of Jesus of Nazareth, how God anointed Him with the Holy Spirit and with power, and how He went about doing good and **healing all who were oppressed by the devil**, for God was with Him. - Acts 10:38 NASB

It's so simple and yet for generations we've failed to connect the dots. Where did sin originate? With that rebellious archangel we now call the devil, satan, the enemy, the serpent. Sin is of the devil, so death is from the devil; sickness and disease are trying to kill you; therefore, sickness and disease are from the devil. Period. And everything of the devil, Jesus came to destroy. This is why Jesus "healed them all." Yes, that's right — Jesus came to destroy your diseases.

Sin brought death into this world — they are conjoined twins, different sides of the same coin, fused. We could not and would not have received death without sin! Sickness, disease and aging (decay) are incipient death. Dying, we shall die. But if sin and sickness are conjoined twins, then so must healing and the remission of sins be!

> He forgives all my sins and heals all my diseases.
> - Psalm 103:3 NLT

> But I want you to know that the Son of Man has authority on earth to forgive sins." So he said to the man, "I tell you, get up, take your mat and go home." He got up, took his mat and walked out in full view of them all. This amazed everyone and they praised God, saying, "We have never seen anything like this!" - Mark 2:10-12 NIV

See how healing and forgiveness are inseparable? The Greek word *iaomai* is defined as:
1. Heal or cure
2. To free from errors or sin, to bring about one's salvation

It is translated into English as *heal* in the accounts of the centurion, the woman with the issue of blood, the epileptic boy, the woman whose daughter was possessed, in "He has sent me to heal the brokenhearted" (Luke 4:18), in "the power of the Lord was present to heal them" (Luke 5:17), and numerous other passages — a total of thirty times in the KJV New Testament. Verse after verse address sin and sickness together or healing and forgiveness together. You'll start to notice that now if you hadn't been aware of it before.

> **If Sin Is Never God's Will, Then Sickness Is Never God's Will**

Our Salvation

> He personally carried our sins in His body on the Cross [willingly offering Himself on it, as on an altar of sacrifice], so that we might die to sin [becoming immune from the penalty and power of sin] and live for righteousness; for by His wounds you [who believe] have been healed.
> - 1 Peter 2:24 AMP

> Surely He has borne our griefs (sicknesses, weaknesses, and distresses) and carried our sorrows and pains [of punishment], yet we [ignorantly] considered Him stricken, smitten, and afflicted by God [as if with leprosy]. But He was wounded for our transgressions, He was bruised for our guilt and iniquities; the chastisement [needful to obtain] peace and well-being for us was upon Him, and with the stripes [that wounded] Him we are healed and made whole.
> - Isaiah 53:4-5 AMPC

> Christ redeemed us from the curse of the law, having become a curse for us; for it is written, cursed is every one that hangeth on a tree. - Galatians 3:13 ASV

> He shall see [the fruit] of the travail of His soul and be satisfied; by His knowledge of Himself [which He possesses and imparts to others] shall My [uncompromisingly] righteous One, My Servant, justify many and make many righteous (upright and in right standing with God), for He

shall bear their iniquities and their guilt [**with the consequences**, says the Lord]. - Isaiah 53:11 AMPC

Did you read the scriptures above, or did you skip down to this line? All of them? Just checking, because, you know, you can't start taking God at His word, or His Word at face value, if you don't read it.

Everything Jesus went through, He endured so that we don't have to. That's why Isaiah 53 is called the substitutionary chapter, and it's why Jesus is called our Substitutionary Sacrifice. God is triune — three unified personages. He created you the same. You are spirit, you have a soul (mind, will and emotions) and you live in a body. Examining verse 5 of Isaiah 53, you'll see that God addressed every aspect of our beings at Calvary, not only our spirits.

Salvation Is a Package Deal

Spirit:
"He was wounded for our transgressions, He was bruised for our iniquities: ..."
- Transgress - to contravene the law
- *Wounded* - translated *pierced* in *Young's Literal Translation* and some others – the shedding of blood for the remission of sins
- Bruising is bleeding **below the surface**— He was likely beaten repeatedly throughout His ordeal
- *Iniquity* - state of immorality, our sin nature, a heart attitude of willfulness against God, original sin – unseen, **below the surface** – Jesus' blood shed under the skin for the cleansing of our sin state (He thinks of everything.)
- Jesus' death - payment in full for the remission of original and fleshly sin, making us righteous in His eyes so that we may have eternal life in heaven, accomplished on the cross

Soul:
"The chastisement for our peace was upon Him, ..."
- Soul - our mind, will & emotions
- He provided peace in every circumstance, joy unspeakable even when facing huge obstacles, and the mind of Christ, His wisdom, all knowledge
- Accomplished in the Garden of Gethsemane when Jesus sweat blood and, knowing what was coming, submitted His will to the Father's; also, throughout His ordeal as He was continually

humiliated, so that we could be esteemed by God; some also attribute benefits to the soul to the crown of thorns

Body:
"And by His stripes we are healed."
- Our physical bodies - healing & divine health provided by His scourging
- Accomplished at the whipping post

Jesus doesn't do anything halfway. He covered every part of our existence — spirit, soul, body. By this *triune* perspective alone, it should be obvious that physical health was provided during Jesus' Passion. We need to amend our definition of *salvation*. According to Isaiah, it's not just eternal life, and he should know — he was pretty tight with the Father.

Salvation is translated from the word *sozo* in Greek, the original language of the New Testament. *Sozo* is a verb (as in, I am saved by grace through faith.) The noun form (as in, I accepted salvation), is the word *soteria*. *Sozo* and *soteria* are surely two of the most important words in all of the Bible, so it's crucial that you have a thorough understanding of them.

From www.preceptaustin.org: "Salvation is a broader term in Greek than we often think of in English. Other concepts that are inherent in *soteria* include restoration to a state of safety, soundness, health and well-being, as well as, preservation from danger of destruction."

William Barclay, theologian and commentator of *The Daily Study Bible* writes: "In classical Greek, *soteria* means 'deliverance' or 'preservation'. It can be used for a man's safe return to his own home or his own country after an absence and a journey. It can mean a 'guarantee of safety' or a 'security against danger'. In the papyri, by far the commonest meaning of soteria is 'bodily health'. For instance, a member of the family writes home, 'Write me a letter about your soteria,' or, as we would say, 'Let me know how you are.'"

And best yet, from www.rockofoffence.com: "The Greek root word associated with the English word salvation is '*sozo*', and it carries several different meanings depending on its use. Some scholars warn that *sozo* or salvation (as used in the Bible) isn't just about "being saved from Hell," but also means: rescue, escape from judgment, deliverance, being preserved from harm, escaping temptation (avoiding sin), renewing the mind, prosperity—and physical healing from sickness and disease (this is not an exhaustive list). For example: **Jesus healed the sick whenever He preached the gospel as an expression of what His salvation provides.**"

Wow. God's Truth is always better than we think. It's too good to be true, yet it is. This is why you have to receive so much of it as personal revelation because worldliness, all the years of living in this natural world, tends to prevent you from believing that any news could be THIS good, or that God wants you to have good things you know you don't deserve. And I'm focusing only on the healing aspects of Jesus' finished work. There's much more that I'll address in future books. Meanwhile, let's continue with the scriptural proof that healing IS contained in Jesus' redemptive work.

I have a question for you. Is there anything further required on Jesus' part to get us into heaven? He died to take the punishment of our sins, so it is finished, right? I'm asking you to wrack your brain, search your heart, and conclude right now that there is nothing else needful on Jesus' part for you to have access to heaven, above and beyond His taking every one of your sins upon Himself and dying in your place of punishment for them. I'm not talking about your part, which is believing, but Jesus' part. Was there anything else He had to do? Is there anything else He has yet to do to pay your way into heaven?

> ### If It's Too Good, It's God

No. He died in your place. The wages of sin is death. It's done.

I was meditating on this, when God revealed to me a profoundly simple truth in the form of a question: "Then why did Jesus volunteer to go through all that other stuff?" That other *stuff* was public humiliation, his beard being ripped from His face, a crown of razor-sharp thorns being smashed down onto his head, and scourging with a cat-o'-nine-tails until the bones of his back were exposed. Why did He submit himself to all that when His death could have been so much easier? Even death by crucifixion, without all the other torture and humiliation, would have been relatively easier, and would still have accomplished opening heaven to us as our eternal home.

Put in graphic modern terms, if you could get your child into heaven for eternity by being beheaded, would you volunteer to first be waterboarded, shocked by a car battery, have your fingernails pulled out, be beaten with a split bamboo cane, have teeth extracted without Novocain, and THEN be led naked to your beheading all to accomplish the same outcome a simple beheading would have produced? Why did Jesus voluntarily go through all that? There had to have been a reason for it.

The Bible clearly answers that question, and you know the answer. In your spirit, you've known it for a very long time.

...by whose stripes ye were healed. - 1Peter 2:24 KJV

Don't waste what He did for you.

Isaiah vs The Apostles on Healing

> Surely He hath borne our griefs, and carried our sorrows…But He was wounded for our transgressions…
> - Isaiah 53:4-5 KJV

The word translated as *griefs* here is the Hebrew *choliy:* sickness. *Mak'ob* is the Hebrew translated as *sorrows*. It means pain (physical) or pain (mental). That's pretty clear, don't you think?

Many times, you'll see Old Testament scriptures referred to or quoted in the New Testament. You can think of that as God's own commentary on those Old Testament verses. Compare these two:

Old Testament:

> Yet he himself bore our sicknesses, and he carried our pains; but we in turn regarded him stricken, struck down by God, and afflicted. But he was pierced because of our rebellion, crushed because of our iniquities; Punishment for our peace was on him, and we are healed by his wounds.
> - Isaiah 53:4-5 CSB

New Testament:

> He himself bore our sins in his body on the tree; so that, having died to sins, we might live for righteousness. By his wounds you have been healed. - 1 Peter 2:24 CSB

Isaiah says you *are* healed, whereas, Peter says you *have been* healed, or *were* healed in some translations. Have you ever wondered about that small difference between the Old and New Testaments? I did, and the answer is so simple and so obvious I can't believe it took me so long to realize it. Isaiah is prophetic, whereas 1 Peter refers to your healing in past tense. Jesus had already done it. The cross was in the past by then. It had already been accomplished when the book of 1 Peter was written, so it's already accomplished now.

Then why are we always trying to GET healing? I can assure you Jesus isn't coming back to do it all over again because you just got a bad report from the doctor. It's already done. He already paid for it. He already provided it.

The scriptures are clear: you were healed two thousand years ago when Jesus, the King of kings and Lord of lords, Creator of the Universe, volunteered to be whipped, to have the flesh of His back ripped off by hooks and jagged bits of metal, even exposing his ribs. The Gospels tell how Jesus went silently, like a lamb to slaughter. Had he said, "Stop!" or "No!" thousands of angels would have swooped down to rescue Him. He said no man could take His life, only He could give it. He was not murdered — He volunteered to take our punishment and forgive our sins. Can you imagine loving anyone so much that you could volunteer for and endure the torture He went through, when a single word could have stopped it? That's what He did for you. It's heartbreaking to contemplate what He went through to spend eternity with you, so that you can be healed, to make your way prosperous in every area of life, to bless you. When I think of that, I want to live for Him, bless Him, obey Him, tell others how wonderful He is.

> By Trying to 'GET' Healing, You're Saying It's Not Yours
>
> Know That It Already Is

Early on in the research for this book, I looked up the word *healed* in Isaiah 53:5 just to be sure that I wasn't relying on second-hand information. I was glad to see it was the Hebrew *rapha*, which I was already familiar with. It means to heal, to make healthful, and it's uses refer to physicians, to healers and most often to being healed by God. According to *Strong's Concordance*, the literal translation of *rapha* is "to mend by stitching", and the practical use is "to cure, cause to heal, physician (treatment), repair and make whole."

That's great news! He made one hundred percent physical wholeness available to you at the cross. It's one of God's names, you know — Jehovah Rapha, the Lord who heals you. I really like *mend by stitching*. To me, that illustrates that it's not only illness Jesus addressed on the cross, but wounds and broken bones. Fast, even instant, healing is available to you if you believe.

Now look again at Peter and Isaiah.
- He has borne our pains of punishment / we are healed
  - Isaiah 53:4-5
- He bore our sin in His own body / you have been healed
  - 1 Peter: 2:24
- He bore our iniquities and guilt / He took the consequences
  - Isaiah 53:11

It was all one transaction. No sin equals no sickness or death. When you deal with the root cause of something, its consequences are no longer an issue, they can no longer come to fruition. We have physical healing because Jesus took our sin. Once we get this into our thick skulls, we don't have to be sick ever again!

No Root = No Fruit

Just as Jesus cursed the fig tree by stating it would no longer bear fruit, and it withered from the roots up; so His dealing with all sin for all time curses the fruit of that sin, which is death. In our day-to-day life, that death comes in the form of sickness and disease and anything that does not promote life, both spiritually and physically. Jesus dealt with sin, paying the price to free you from its physical and spiritual fruit.

Remember the passage in Matthew that you read in "Chapter 1 - Jesus Came to Execute God's Will"?

> ...and healed all who were sick, that it might be fulfilled which was spoken by Isaiah the prophet, saying: "He Himself took our infirmities and bore our sicknesses."
> - Matthew 8:17 NKJV

This verse irreversibly ties Isaiah to the New Testament passages and states categorically that 1 Peter and Isaiah both are referring to PHYSICAL healing. He *healed all who were sick* to fulfill Isaiah's prophecy – *He hath borne our griefs* (sicknesses), *and carried our sorrows* (physical and mental pain). You can never again say that Jesus' stripes were for spiritual healing. He healed sick people's bodies to fulfill Isaiah's prophecies!

But Wait, There's More...

Even though I keep showing you scriptures that are NOT referring to spiritual healing, I don't want us to forget the spiritual benefits. They ARE more important in the long run. Our Lord went through horrific spiritual agonies when He took each person on earth's sin. He even went to hell for us, where He conquered that realm and took back the keys to our dominion.

Jesus had never before felt the guilt or shame of a single transgression or wayward thought. He took all our anxiety, depression, feelings of inadequacy, broken hearts, every mental disease and distress and our difficulty subduing our flesh. He paid for all the harassments of our souls.

Now we can have the peace that surpasses all understanding that the Holy Spirit wants to share with us.

He took all that — saving our spirit man, our soul, and our physical body, our entire triune being, two thousand years ago, in one COMPLETE and FINISHED work. The physical torture was for saving our physical bodies — for our health. How can you live the abundant life Jesus said He came to bring you if you're not healthy? How can you go on mission trips if you're not robust? How can you be a shining example to the world of how good our God is if you're sickly? How can you teach Sunday School when you're afraid you'll spread your cold to the children?

We can now see that disease, sickness and aging (with its *normal* symptoms of failing eyesight and hearing, aches and pains) are all a result of sin in this world. They are not *normal* for citizens of the Kingdom of God (that's you!). You have received the gift of righteousness, so these sin consequences no longer apply to you.

Jesus came to restore God's plan, to reverse the curse, to undo everything satan had accomplished on this earth, to make everything right again as the second and final Adam. Every good thing destroyed by sin and the consequences of the resulting curse has been returned to its original form and intent, **legally and in the spiritual realm**, by Jesus' work at the cross, for those who accept Him. (See Genesis 3:16-19 and Deuteronomy 28:1-14.) It has been accomplished legally, so every good thing is again available to us as believers.

Two thousand years ago, the Jews really understood the whole atonement thing. They'd been making sacrifices in return for blessings for generations. If something bad happened to you, it was because you had sinned since the last acceptable sacrifice.

> Sin = Sickness
> Therefore
> Forgiveness = Health

So when they heard that Jesus had been the one sacrifice for all time, they understood instantly — all-encompassing blessings were now theirs. They got it! The New Covenant in Jesus' blood was the best thing since manna. The man born crippled is a great example. This man heard Paul preach on the forgiveness of sin and the gospel of grace. By accepting that forgiveness, he understood he was now righteous in the eyes of Jehovah, and therefore, there was no sin to be atoned for by his deformity. Paul perceived that the man had received that revelation and, therefore, had faith for healing (Acts 14:9). So he told the man to get up and walk, and the man sprang up and danced a jig. (I'm paraphrasing, but isn't that what your reaction would be?)

Sin and sickness are one. Forgiveness and healing are one. According to the Gospel — which the church is NOT preaching — when you get saved, you get healed. I wish I'd known that at the time. How about you?

PART TWO
Remember the Great Things He Has Done

I will tell of the loving kindnesses of the Lord, and the praiseworthy deeds of the Lord, according to all that the Lord has done for us… - Isaiah 63:7 AMP

[Earnestly] remember the former things, [which I did] of old; for I am God, and there is no one else; I am God, and there is none like Me - Isaiah 46:9 AMP

One generation will commend Your works to the next, and they shall proclaim your mighty acts, the glorious splendor of Your majesty. And I will meditate on Your wondrous works. - Psalm 145:4,5 BSB

And they overcame him by the blood of the Lamb and by the word of their testimony - Revelation 12:11 KJV

Therefore many other signs Jesus also performed in the presence of the disciples, which are not written in this book; but these have been written so that you may believe that Jesus is the Christ, the Son of God; and that believing you may have life in His name. - John 20:30-31 NASB

CHAPTER 4
As You Believe, So Be It

Why would I take the time and go to the Herculean effort to write and publish this book just to convince you that God heals today? Why would I care what you believe?

- Because God cares. He wrote so much about healing in the Bible that it's obviously important to Him. It's important to Him because He loves each of us so very much.
- Because healing is an evangelical tool. It's been called the dinner bell to salvation. It's the number one reason people seek God.
- Because God wants us hale and hearty. He has called us to good works, and a healthy body makes more of those works possible.
- Because of compassion. You read in the Bible that Jesus was *moved with compassion* to heal the multitudes. So compassion, the deep, undeniable desire to relieve suffering, is another primary motivation.
- Because healing defeats the enemy, demolishes his works, and proves to everyone that he's a liar.

For these reasons I want you to avail yourself of the healing Jesus purchased for you, and they are also reasons you should want to be healed.

Why do we sing songs about our mighty God, all-powerful, our defender, when we've never given Him a chance to show us that is Who He is? We're singing about the God of the Bible, not proclaiming our personal, living God, our best friend, the One Whose lovingkindness and demonstrable miracles we can live expecting daily.

As a young child, I was flipping through television channels one night and was halted by curiosity about what was happening on the screen. A man in a suit put his hand on the forehead of another man, causing him to fall. Just a touch, and the man collapsed! I remember thinking he was lucky there happened to be somebody behind him to catch him. As it turned out, the man in the suit had been praying for the other man. He was praying for other people, too. And he was saying that they were healed of whatever was wrong with each one. I'd never heard of that before. I yelled, "Mama, c'mere — hurry."

I pointed to the screen and waited a moment while she listened and watched. "Is that real?"

She had that expression parents get when they don't want to answer their kid's question, especially when they don't know the answer. "Well... the church we belong to doesn't believe in that."

Huh. That wasn't a response I'd anticipated. I'd asked a yes-or-no question, hadn't I? I tried to digest what she'd said for a moment, but couldn't quite figure out how it qualified as an answer. "But is it real?"

"The church we belong to doesn't believe in it."

At least she was consistent. That was the only answer I could get out of her.

What I admire to this day is that Mom refused to take the party line and say, "No." Even raised as a Methodist and attending First Baptist in a small southern town since marriage, she was careful not to put God in a box of man's making. My mom's a pretty smart cookie, as they said back then.

That was a sleepless night for this child full of questions, but it led, years hence, to this book you're reading now. I knew that very night that if it was real, when I grew up, I wanted to touch people and see them healed.

To me, God's the One Who raised MY child back to life, Who physically transported ME to make possible something important to ME, Who healed ME of the incurable and deadly, Who multiplies MY finances. He is MY Heavenly Father, MY ever-present help. He's not distant. He's MY God. I am the one He loves. Am I being selfish? Was I selfish to expect my husband or my dad to love me? I expected good things from them because I trusted in their love for me. How much more does my Father in heaven love me? He delights in doing good things for me. He loves to surprise me, the same way I enjoy surprising those I love with good things.

How could I not want **you** to know God this way when I know He wants to do the same for you? Your being blessed by God is not going to mean there's less for me — His riches are endless. If you don't experience God in these ways — healing you, surprising you with good things, constantly blessing you in every area — it's only because you don't believe He wants to move in these ways. But I promise you He does.

King David advises us to encourage OURSELVES in the Lord, remembering all the great things He has done (Psalms 77 & 105). You can express this as entering His gates with thanksgiving and His courts with praise (Psalm 100). When you're in need, there's no better advice because remembering those past victories in Him and His goodness and love for you raises the level of your faith and confidence in Him. That's the David Principle at work. If you can't think of anything to praise Him for, here's a reminder: Jesus and breath.

Back when I was a child, I noticed some bumper stickers around town printed with "Expect a Miracle!" I found out the quote came from some preacher named Oral Roberts, but I didn't hear that at First Baptist. I heard it from a childhood friend whose family was considered a little *out there* by Baptist standards. Well, one day many years later, I took the advice of those bumper stickers, and life has been an exciting adventure ever since. He does more than you can ask or even imagine. I found this first paragraph of an Oral Roberts sermon in the ministry's online archives (used with permission).

> "Miracles were always happening in the Bible because people were expecting them to happen. They were looking for them to happen. They were believing God for them to happen. People expected God to stretch out His mighty hand and display His supernatural power in their lives. They opened their hearts to His miracle-working power, and miracles happened!"

Expectation Is the Highest Form of Faith

Carlie Terradez from Colorado Springs (*http://terradezministies.com*) says of the church she belonged to in England before she was healed of epilepsy, "Our faith worked perfectly. We got exactly what we believed for, every time — which was nothing." The point: your beliefs determine your expectations, and your expectations yield results. So, as your beliefs change by the power of the Word and the Holy Spirit, you get better and better results.

Let it happen, then, just as you believe! - Matthew 9:29 GN

Go! As you have believed, so will it be done for you.
- Matthew 8:13 GN

It's your responsibility to do the work to get your beliefs in line with God's word. This is called renewing your mind. And it is **SO** worth the effort. You have to establish God's goodness deep in your heart in order to have faith and an intimate relationship with Him. You can start that process by reminding yourself of things God has already done for you. Number one on the list: He sent Jesus.

Before we examine some of the beliefs (in Part 4) that keep us from God's will being accomplished in our bodies, I want to share with you a few personal examples of divine healing in this day and age — **proof** He heals today. Keep in mind that these (and more) occurred over a period of perhaps twenty years, at different levels of my knowledge and faith regarding healing.

CHAPTER 5
Real-Life Examples

Cured of the Incurable

"I've never seen anybody this bad. It's going to kill you, and it's going to kill you soon!" That's what the sleep lab technician told me after the obvious diagnosis of sleep apnea. I was waking myself up every five seconds to take a breath, and the tech told me he'd never seen a case as bad as mine. There was no cure, only the CPAP machine that creates positive air pressure to keep your airway from collapsing while you sleep. It was my only hope, he said.

Three years I'd gone without a decent night's sleep. It affected every area of my life. I could fall asleep on the dais during church, in front of everyone. Driving was a nightmare. Needless to say my temper was short, and my relationships with my husband and my son were suffering. I remember asking the Lord to remove my rage, lying that I'd read my Bible every day if He did. (Note to all: God doesn't need or want you to try to earn his blessings.) He took the rage, but I'm not going to tell you how many days in a row I read my Bible before failing grossly.

As to the sleep apnea, I craved junk food for instant energy, and became addicted to drive-thrus. I would drive fifteen miles to a pick-up window rather than make something healthy at home. That addiction led to more health problems. I really had no idea how much the apnea was impacting my life, because it had become my normal.

I gave the CPAP machine my best shot, even praying for help from heaven, but the dry air burned my mouth and throat, and the mask made me claustrophobic. I finally couldn't keep the panic down, and came up out of the bed clawing that mask off.

"You HAVE to wear this!" The tech was truly concerned, but I knew somebody that could fix me without any machine.

> Trust in the LORD with all your heart, And lean not on your own understanding. - Proverbs 3:5 NKJV

The technician didn't have a very supportive response to my faith stance. "Oh don't give me that! My daddy was a Baptist missionary, and I've heard all that before. God helps those that help themselves, and you have to use this CPAP, or you won't live much longer." I wanted to tell him that was a lie from the pit of hell — God wants us to fully rely on Him and *lean not on our own understanding*. Maybe I was just too tired to argue.

"Just call my husband to pick me up, please. Don't worry about me. I'll be healed Sunday morning."

I pulled my pastor aside thirty-two hours later, told her what was going on, and that I wasn't leaving church until I was healed. I'd stay all day, all week if necessary. So at the end of the service, she told everyone I was coming down front for healing and invited anyone that needed healing to join me. The pastor didn't pray over us — we were on our own in front of the Throne of Grace.

I didn't beg God, and I didn't try to make a deal — I'd learned that lesson. To be honest, I wasn't even reverent. I stood at the altar, arms crossed, and took my case to the Creator of the Universe, "The Bible says it was accomplished 2000 years ago, that it's Your will. If the Bible says it, You said it, and it's impossible for You to lie. So You don't have any choice but to heal me right now. I'm writing a check on my heavenly account as a joint heir with Christ for healing of sleep apnea. I'm coming boldly before your throne, and I'm not leaving until I know I'm healed."

By the time I felt my lungs open up, everyone else had left the altar. I don't know about them, but I was healed. I was cured of the incurable. Who can do that? Nobody but the Living God. And He loves you just as much as He loves me.

Did I really have to wait until Sunday morning to receive my healing? No. It just seemed like the easiest way, with my support system lifting me up in prayer and wonderful music to carry me into the throne room. But could I have gone into prayer or praise alone with the same results? Absolutely. You can receive your healing right now, right where you are, reading this book on a bus headed in to work, in the hospital, in bed at night with your spouse bugging you to turn off the light, or at the beach with the sun that God created just for you pounding down.

I'm still kicking myself, though, for not asking for more that Sunday morning. So ask big.

Want more examples? No problem. I have lots...an entire book full, in fact. (No idea when that one will be published.)

Kevin's Leg – Healed

Honeymooning in the hospital is not ideal. But Kevin needed a skin graft before he could return to work as a ship's officer. A plastic surgeon we'd just met came to our room after the scheduled skin graft, and said he couldn't complete the surgery because there was nothing to graft to. Kevin had already had multiple surgeries to repair shattered bones just above his left ankle, and infection had eaten away at his flesh, underneath the cast they'd just removed. By the time the surgeon had debrided the wound (cleaned all the dead tissue out), there was a 1x4 inch hole all the way down to the bone. Well, to the vitallium plate that was supposed to be strengthening the tibia. And there was a red line running up Kevin's leg due to that infection — osteomyelitis.

We'd been married one week when we were told Kevin's leg had to be amputated or he would die.

Short version: six weeks living in Baptist Hospital in Pensacola, intravenous Vancomycin burning out his veins, and still that red line advanced. Neither of us had gone to church for years by then, but you can bet I was praying — praying desperate prayers with muscles tense, teeth gritted, brow furrowed, tears escaping. Every evening, the doctor would stop by on his rounds, pull out sterilized tools, pull back the last layer of bandaging and tap-tap-tap with the surgical steel probe on the vitallium plate. "No change yet." Every evening. For six weeks. Forty-two days. No change except that the red line got longer.

I was renewing Kevin's bandage every six hours, as the nurses thought it best to keep me busy and involved. Something I couldn't quite put my finger on changed in the look of that gaping wound one day. Six hours later I called in the nurse. Kevin saw the curious look on her face, but there wasn't enough change to say anything aloud. Another six hours passed and I called the nurse in again. There was no doubt now. The wound was changing. Flesh was growing in. Six hours later, every nurse on the floor gathered to see. That wound was closing so rapidly it made me think of watching time lapse photography of a flower bud opening, in reverse.

The doctor had emergency surgery that evening, so missed his rounds. But the next night, he pulled out the probe and tried to tap between the staples, but the probe wouldn't go in. The red line had vanished. "What are you two still doing here? Haven't you gone home yet?" I burst into tears. Before he left our room, he turned back and told us, "I had nothing to do with this healing — this wasn't me."

God gives more than you can ask or think though, so there is more to this story. When my mother was a girl, my grandparents had borrowed from my great grandfather to buy a big chunk of an island that had been created by a hurricane — Santa Rosa Island. My grandfather participated in the development of that island, on which flourished Pensacola Beach and the town of Gulf Breeze. After surgery and six weeks of care, the bill from our plastic surgeon was nearly zero. He'd found out that my grandparents had donated the land his church was built on. Thank you, Doctor – you know who you are.

Kevin's Leg – Restored
A Creative Miracle

Eleven years later, but still before we rededicated our lives to the Lord, Kevin had back surgery, made necessary by having lost an inch and a half off the length of that leg when the bones were reconstructed. The surgeon was wonderful; the results for Kevin's back were great. But the leg length still had to be addressed to reduce the chance of further back issues. So Kevin had to put a small lift into his shoes, and buy shoes with the type of soles that could be ripped off and modified.

Ships and the chemicals on deck can cause rapid degradation of shoe soles, and Kevin would often get to the end of his time at home and realize his shoes were at the point that they might not make it through another month shipboard, so last-minute shopping commenced. For years, before every two or three trips to work on his ship, we'd spend the last couple of days running around town looking for runner-type shoes that were not constructed with integrated soles, and they became harder and harder to find as fashions evolved. Then we'd have to search out a shoe repair person to pull the sole off and install a one-inch wedge, as a rush job.

Meanwhile, we both got born again. One day, I got mad, realizing this was a way that the enemy was stealing from us! He was stealing our time, our peace and our money. Our time together those last couple of days before Kevin departed for another 36 days of work and travel should have been spent having fun and quality time together as a family, not running around stores and inhaling shoe glue fumes. And the money was no small part of the issue either. So yes, I got angry at the enemy. I wasn't going to stand for that any more. He'd overplayed his hand. I'd seen through the everyday occurrences and realized he was at the root of this theft, and it wasn't happening again.

Shortly afterward, while Kevin was still at sea, I was walking through a store to get to an appointment in the mall wearing imaginary blinders so I wouldn't see things I'd be tempted to spend money on. But one thing did catch my attention. I kept walking. Then the Lord arrested me, and I turned around. There on a rack was the sexiest pair of men's driving mocs I'd ever seen, on clearance, in Kevin's size. Mocs cannot have the sole altered. They were perfect.

Kevin arrived home the day of an evangelist friend's spiritual warfare seminar. I rushed him home from the airport for a shower, then we were out the door to get to the church on time. "Stop! What're you wearing?!

You're supposed to wear those driving mocs tonight as evidence of your faith. Why are you wearing your work shoes?"

"I'll be walking in circles if I don't have my lifts. I'll wear the driving mocs after."

"You're only walking from the parking lot into the church. It won't kill you to limp that far."

After the seminar, the presenter was leaving. "Jimmy, don't forget about Kevin's leg — it needs growing out."

"Oh, right! Kevin, have a seat. Make sure your back is flat against the chair back, legs straight out, toes up, so we can see the difference in lengths. This is the easiest thing in the world to pray for."

The difference in Kevin's legs was obvious. As Jimmy prayed a quick, simple prayer, telling that left leg what to do, I watched in amazement as the left heel just seemed to shift downward until it was perfectly even with the right one.

"Awesome!" I said. "Now, could you add about four inches to both legs?"

Trial by Fire – Mom's Arm

The call came from my grandmother. "No need for you to leave work, but you should know, your mother was in a wreck..."

Ten minutes later I burst through the laundry room door, then nearly turned and ran out again, because from the other end of the house I could hear my mom moaning in pain. She handled pain well, so I couldn't even imagine what she was going through.

The station wagon had burst into flames with my mother inside, and her upper left arm had been burned badly before she'd gotten out. Her income came from being a church musician and teaching piano, but the doctor said she'd never play again.

I couldn't stay and listen to that, so I made an excuse to my dad and came back an hour or so later, with my mind better prepared to cope with what was, as a teenager, a very disturbing circumstance. As I entered through that same door into the darkened laundry room, I was startled by a moving shadow. It was my mother sorting laundry!

"What are you doing up?! You're...you're...supposed to be..."

"I'm better now." I didn't know it at the time, but later saw that she had a way of getting in the zone with God and flowing in His healing when the situation was desperate.

A week later, she was teaching, and the following Sunday she was back at the church organ. She's eighty now, and just put in her retirement notice... but not due to failing health.

The Easiest Thing to Pray For
Passing it On

God does not waste our experiences. He turns them all, good and bad, to ultimate good for us, and for others. Is your healing only for yourself? No, just as He gives you financial blessings so that you can bless others, He heals you and proves to others He still heals today. Like anything else, it's easier to have faith for healing when you've experienced or witnessed healing yourself. (Thomas wasn't the only doubter.)

I had done it before, laid on hands and seen healing occur, but it was usually with a group. On one occasion, the person we were praying over was healed and said that she knew it from the heat coming off my hands when I touched her. Interestingly, her healing was for a problem she had at the location of my hands, but not for the condition that I was praying for!

The day came, though, when it all fell into place. A man had asked for ministry from my cell group. When we were just talking, visiting, getting to know him, he mentioned he had one leg shorter than the other, and it was causing some back problems. Sound familiar? I knew I had finally met my now-or-never moment. If I wasn't obedient in that moment, my ministry would die before it was born.

I jumped up, repeating what Jimmy had said before praying over Kevin's leg, "That's the easiest thing in the world to pray for." I commanded his leg, and watched it grow out before my eyes. Then I burst into tears. He joined my friends in surrounding me in a group hug as I recovered from that emotional moment remembering my husband and praising God for using me to pass on what He had done for Kevin years before.

So when you have read this book, go forth in Jesus' Name, lay hands on the sick, and they shall recover.

STAND YOUR GROUND
Authority in Action

Testimony from Shontesha Price, guest author:

Back in December 2018, we had just arrived home from a family vacation. When we got inside we found pools of water sitting in the floor all over the house. It came to our knowledge that our hot water tank malfunctioned, shot water out over into our boiler which was near it and caused it to send out steam instead of heat. Wow! A restoration team had to come and dry out the walls with these special machines and put solution down. All kinds of stuff was done to get the house right, including tearing some of the rooms down and completely rebuilding them. The company said it was safe to live there while all this was going on even though I was a little skeptical about it. One day I woke up, and I felt congested and stuffy, tickly and tingly. It progressed, and I felt horrible. But it seemed I only felt that way in my bedroom. By this time I was full of mucus. Man, did I feel bad. And yes, I was praying, but I wasn't getting any relief. So, I decided to sleep in my living room, and I felt better. The second night, same thing. By the 3rd night, that was it!!! I was fed up!!!! No more!! I'd been run out of my own bed, couldn't sleep with my husband, house a mess, sick. I wasn't going to take it. I told satan to TAKE IT BACK!!! If it ain't good and perfect, it's from the enemy! While every sickness is not a demon, satan is the root of all sickness. It entered the earth when Adam and Eve sinned against God. This daughter of Abraham was not going to take it. As long as you're willing to tolerate sickness or anything else that's not God's best, you will. You'll live with it because you can still function. Functioning, but yet not living an abundant life, is a trap to remain in the condition you're currently in. Don't do it. Bust out!

I stood on the passage of scripture in 2 Chronicles Chapter 20. The whole chapter came to mind. Jehoshaphat prayed and depended on God for their deliverance. He began by boasting on how big and mighty our God is, that there is no power on earth or anywhere greater than His. Then he reminded God of the covenant He had made with Abraham. He didn't stop there! He remembered His father's prayer that he prayed over the people at the dedication of the temple, asking God to answer the people when they cried out to Him. Holy Spirit made Jehoshaphat's prayer come alive inside of me that night in my living room. I thought of the covenant I have with God, sealed by the blood of Jesus, with faith in that Name. How dare satan offend the covenant that I have with my God — a covenant that's greater than Abraham's and all the saints of the Old Testament! Healing belongs to me. I'm an heir of salvation. My Father would never want this for me. He paid a price for it, His son, my Lord, Jesus Christ!! Satan tried to drive me out of my bed with my husband and to trespass and illegally step foot on God's property. Yes, I'm His property. He is mine and I am His!

I took my authority, exercised my rights as a citizen and ambassador of the Kingdom of God and commanded sickness to leave my body! Oh, and I didn't say it very sweetly and nicely. I spoke with authority and I meant business. I told satan to take it back. Get out of my body now!! I felt the mucus start to dry up from my nose all the way to the back of my throat. My nasal passages popped open, and I could breathe. Every symptom I had left my body in seconds. And I felt it leave, and satan came and did exactly what I said. He took his sickness back because it does not belong to me! I refuse to pay for something Jesus has already paid for.

We as God's children can live in divine health. The key is to submit to God, resist the devil, and he will flee. He doesn't have a choice except to back up off of us. Refuse to accept sickness and disease, nor tolerate it, nor function in it. Choose to be free!! At the first sign of a symptom know that our Father does not want to see you suffer in any way, shape or form. He loves us. Jesus has given us His authority and name to trample over all the powers of the enemy. Don't allow anything to hurt you! Be free!!!

Using her authority as a believer, Shontesha has banished twenty-three chronic symptoms from her body. Learn more about employing the authority Jesus granted you in Shontesha's new book *TALK BACK*. Wait until you read about God telling her to command the sun — it'll blow your mind! You have the same power living inside you that Shontesha has, praise God — it's the same Holy Spirit that Jesus received at His baptism and that raised Him from the dead. Put your authority to work now, and demand the devil and his sickness leave your body.

Part Three
God's Word is True

Give me life in accordance with your faithful love, and I will obey...your word is forever; it is firmly fixed in heaven. ...If your instruction had not been my delight, I would have died in my affliction. - Psalm 119:88-92 CSB

The entirety of Your word *is* truth, And every one of Your righteous judgments *endures* forever.
- Psalm 119:160 NKJV

Now, O Lord God, You are God, and Your words are truth, and You have promised this good thing to Your servant. - 2 Samuel 7:28 ESV

Sanctify them [purify, consecrate, separate them for Yourself, make them holy] by the Truth; Your Word is Truth .- John 17:17 AMPC

God is not a man, that He should lie, or a son of man, that he should change his mind. Has he said, and will he not do it? Or has he spoken and will he not fulfill it? Behold, I have received a command to bless; **He has blessed and I cannot revoke it.** - Numbers 23:19,20 ESV

CHAPTER 6
Why Don't We Take God's Word at Face Value?

Why is it so difficult for us to believe that God's Word means what it says? How is it that we can sit in church and listen to the scriptures being read, say "Amen", read them in our daily devotions, agree with them, yet never see the truth in them or actually put them to work for our own benefit in our day-to-day lives? That's what they're there for, you know. Everything God tells us is for our benefit. So why do we stare at the words on the page and never comprehend that they're real, and they're accurate, and they mean what they say? We don't have that problem when reading science texts. We pretty well swallow whatever they say without question — same with newspapers. But there's a veil over our eyes when it comes to reading the Word of God.

> Yes, even today when they read Moses' writings, their hearts are covered with that veil, and they do not understand. - 2 Corinthians 3:15 NLT

Unfortunately, as discussed in Chapter 3, the problem lies in part with what we've been taught through a lifetime of Sunday School and sermons — doctrinal decrees that are so far removed from God's Truth as to sometimes be the opposite of what the Bible is telling us. Hard to believe? Yes, it is. But, it's nonetheless true. God Himself foreknew this would happen. He stated that our traditions would make His Word of no effect in our lives, and that His people would be destroyed for lack of knowledge of Him.

> You nullify the word of God by your tradition that you have handed down. And you do many other similar things.
> - Mark 7:13 CSB

> He answered them, "Isaiah prophesied correctly about you hypocrites, as it is written: This people honors me with their lips, but their heart is far from me. They worship me in vain, **teaching as doctrines human commands**. Abandoning the command of God, **you hold on to human tradition**." - Mark 7: 6-8 CSB

> My people are destroyed for lack of knowledge: because thou hast rejected knowledge… - Hosea 4:6 KJV

Did you realize that the second part of that scripture (Hosea 4:6) says it's because we have *REJECTED knowledge*? We need to take a close look at the teachings we've heard all our lives, and determine if they're accurate or if they're holding us back from receiving the truths the Lord wants to pour into us. Which of the lessons you learned and the sermons you listened to have been twisted by the enemy into subtle deceptions? Let's go on a precept-busting adventure.

We're in good company — even Paul was in this position. As a learned Pharisee, he knew all the prophecies about the coming Messiah, yet he walked in unbelief and persecuted anyone who followed Jesus. But when Truth stared him in the face, up close and personal, he could not deny it. That's why this book was written, for you to stare into the face of Truth, in the hope that you will receive this revelation: God wants you and your loved ones healed right now. He wants you to receive His life into your body.

It's so much easier to believe what we believe, to settle for what we have always known, to stay in that comfort zone. But your comfort zone may not be where God is. In fact, He's really not all that wild about comfort zones, is He? He never leaves his people sitting on their laurels. Stagnation is not a mode of operation in the Kingdom of God. He moves, and we're expected to follow. But He also wants us to take initiative.

> Go ye therefore… - Matthew 28:19 KJV

He wants us to KNOW His will and move accordingly to enforce it on the earth — that's what giving us dominion is all about. How do you learn what His will is? Primarily by getting into the Word.

So what if you've heard the same thing over and over all your life, in Sunday School, sermons, books you've read, in Bible college or from professors on the road to your doctorate in theology? None of that makes it true. It only means you've stuck to one doctrinal camp in your studies. Your truth needs to come from the Godhead's mouth.

Ask yourself these questions instead. Have you ever asked God a question and heard an answer during your personal Bible study or deep worship? Have you asked the Holy Spirit to reveal the meaning of a scripture passage to you, and then felt new understanding wash over you? Have you heard the voice of God deep inside? Have you seen the words literally jump off the page and into your soul? Has knowledge that you can

Believe What God Believes Everything Else Is a Lie No Matter How Good It Sounds

barely find words to explain in English fallen into your heart inexplicably when you pressed in to find an answer? Have you ever experienced a physical sensation you've never had before, attached to new understanding? If none of these things accompanied your understanding of God's goodness or divine healing, then question what you believe, because it may be from the understanding of man.

Don't expect these things to happen every time. We're not supposed to go by what we *feel*. It's just that God has a way of letting us know when it's Him you're hearing. Dive deeper. Ask the Father Himself. He loves to answer our questions. Christianity is all about your personal relationship with God. When you hear Truth, you know it in the very fiber of your being. You really need to look more closely at the scriptures and ask the Holy Spirit to reveal the deep truths contained in them regardless of what you've always been taught.

Don't believe me — it's God who says our traditions (historic denominational beliefs) strangle what He has sent the Word to accomplish in our lives. His Word is not returning to Him void. It's accomplishing healing for many people. Please don't miss out. Remember that God's Word is God's Will. His Word says you were healed when Jesus took the scourging. You want to be positioned within His will for you, don't you?

We have all been deceived to some degree — we all have misconceptions about God. We will never know it all, because our subject, the Almighty, is infinite. But you can start by beginning to believe that the Word means what it says. Begin to believe that the scriptures are true! This is essential to eradicating erroneous beliefs you may have unknowingly had for years.

Start in a practical way. Pick any scripture verse about healing that resonates with you. Pray over it. Engage with the Holy Spirit. Read each word slowly, and check the definitions of words to see what depth of meaning you've missed the previous hundred times you read it. Speak it aloud, openly or under your breath, putting emphasis on different words each time. Then read eight or ten verses before and after that passage to get the context. Context is everything. Meditate on it.

> Your righteous testimonies are everlasting and Your Decrees are binding to eternity; give me understanding and I shall live [give me discernment and comprehension and I shall not die]. - Psalm 119:144 AMPC

And here's a free tip to use when reading the Bible: do not make a doctrine out of one verse. Huge errors are made that way. We'll see some examples of that in Part Four.

You're Being Sabotaged!

Before we go any further, let's look at four tendencies of the church today that result in robbing us of the abundant life that scripture tells us God wants us to live. These tendencies skew the way we read the Word, affecting the conclusions we draw and the effectiveness of God's Word in our everyday lives.

Please don't think I'm trying to tear down the church — it is Jesus' bride, and He loves it. But man-made doctrines and practices from the Dark Ages still plague God's church today and must be rooted out if we are to receive what God has always wanted for us and become His spotless bride. Health and godly prosperity SHOULD be byproducts of receiving the gospel (3 John 1:2). Living the Gospel brings persecution, though, so this is not about living a comfortable life. It's about getting to know God personally, which is HIS deepest desire, and about attracting others to Him. As you live life here on earth, every area of your life should shine with God's blessings — from His love to His provision — so that others are drawn in, and receive eternal life, God-given purpose, peace, joy, and all the things that come to believers from above. **You are blessed to be a blessing.**

So here are four ways we look at scripture that sabotage our understanding of God's word.

1. We spiritualize the scriptures.

We tend to apply the Word primarily to eternal arenas rather than to our everyday life here on earth. You need to know which scriptures apply to eternity and which apply to here and now —

> Scripture We Misapply to Heaven Is Useless Here and Now

at this time, particularly as regards your health, because your health affects every area of your life. The scriptures are quite clear if you only take a moment to check the original languages. **The word *life* is probably the biggest stumbling block to our understanding the scriptures accurately.** For this reason, I'm giving you the full definitions here. They are taken directly from *www.biblestudytools.com*.

Zoe — yes, like the girls' name.
1. life
    a. the state of one who is possessed of vitality or is animate animate
    b. every living soul
2. life
    a. of the absolute fullness of life, both essential and ethical, which belongs to God, and through him both to the hypostatic "logos" and to Christ in whom the "logos" put on human nature
    b. life real and genuine, a life active and vigorous, devoted to God, blessed, in the portion even in this world of those who put their trust in Christ, but after the resurrection to be consummated by new accessions (among them a more perfect body), and to last forever.

So the primary definition is life as we think of it here on earth – the fact that we are alive. And the secondary definition speaks to me about the abundant life, blessed through Christ, leading to an amazing eternal life.

Zao is the verb form of *zoe*.
1. to live, breathe, be among the living (not lifeless, not dead)
2. to enjoy real life
    a. to have true life and worthy of the name
    b. active, blessed, endless in the kingdom of God
3. to live, i.e., pass life, in the manner of the living and acting of mortals or character
4. living water, having vital power in itself and exerting the same upon the soul
5. Metaphor - to be in full vigour
    a. to be fresh, strong, efficient,
    b. as adj. active, powerful, efficacious

As you can see, *zoe* and *zao* reference our physical life. Note that when **pointed out specifically**, it can extend into eternal life (definition 2b and 1Timothy 4:8 two paragraphs below), but it always refers first to our physical life here on the earth, and particularly to a good and purposeful life (abundant) life. Eternal life is *zoe aionios*...

> For the wages of sin is death but the free gift of God is eternal life **(zoe aionios)** in Christ Jesus our Lord.
> - Romans 6:23 ESV

Another Greek term for eternal life is used in Timothy. In the verse below, the *life that is now*, is encapsulated in the word *nyn*, and *that which is to come* is the word *mello*. The scripture, again, is specific — zoe now and zoe to come.

> For bodily exercise profiteth little; but goodness is profitable unto all things, having promise of the life that now is, and of that which is to come. - 1 Timothy 4:8 KJV

My point is that scripture makes it clear when it is referring to eternity. **Life means life, *eternal life* means eternal life.** If you want to check every scripture you encounter that contains the word *life*, it's easy to do. Some cell phone Bible apps even include interlinear concordances. But know that when a scripture refers to eternal life, it says *eternal life*. Otherwise, it means our physical, and particularly our abundant life here on this earth.

It amazes me over and over again as I search the scriptures how merciful God is, that even in Old Testament times He wanted to save our physical lives.

> … And I will take sickness away from the midst of you. No one shall suffer miscarriages or be barren in your land; I will fulfill the number of your days. - Exodus 23:35 NKJV

> …for I am the Lord that healeth thee. - Exodus 15:26 KJV

> Behold, I will bring it health and cure, and I will cure them, and will reveal unto them the abundance of peace and truth.
> - Jeremiah 33:6 NKJV

In Ancient Hebrew, the word translated *death* is *maveth*: death, dying, state of death, realm of the dead. That's pretty dead. *Chayah*, the word translated *live* is: to live, to have life, remain alive, to live prosperously, to revive or be quickened (from sickness, discouragement, death). That sounds a lot like abundant life and healing on this earth.

Heaven is good. We'll be eternally happy there. Got it. We really don't need to know much more than that. St. Peter will probably hand out brochures as we pass through the pearly gates. Yes, I'm being silly. But, God placed us on Earth. He even created this planet FOR us. It was His will that we live here. So doesn't it make sense that the Bible, our instruction manual, would tell us more about how to go about life here than it does about our future in Heaven?

2. We forget that God created man to be immortal on this earth.

That's how He created Adam and Eve, immortal and disease-free. Only when sin came in did they begin physically aging and become susceptible to all manner of disease (signs of incipient death, of atrophy and decay, of corruption), and eventually their bodies died. What

> Jesus Reversed the Curse so You Can Now Walk in His Immunity

seems normal to us must have been quite a shock to the first couple. They'd never experienced aches and pains, never expected their eyesight or hearing to diminish, never heard of a cold. None of these things are God's will for us, and we know this because God did not create Adam and Eve with these limitations. He could not have called sickness and disease good. God created everything to be perfect and according to His will. So I'll repeat myself: sickness and disease are not part of God's will for mankind. They entered the world through sin. **Sickness cannot be God's will anymore than sin can.**

3. We don't truly believe that God is no respecter of persons.

What does *no respecter of persons* mean in practical terms? It means He does not show favoritism — He loves us all equally. He tells us that He makes no differentiation between people. If He does it for one, He'll do it for every single one of us. In fact, He DID it for every single one of us. We only have to believe that, know that, expect that.

> Opening his mouth, Peter said: "I most certainly understand now that God is not one to show partiality, but in every nation the man who fears Him and does what is right is welcome to Him. - Acts 10:34,35 NASB

> For God does not show favoritism. - Romans 2:11 BSB
>
> "Yet He is not partial to princes, nor does He regard the rich more than the poor; for they are all the work of His hands." - Job 34:19 NKJV

Are you *the work of His hands*? If He did it for one person, He will do it for you. He has to! Why? Because He has made a point of telling us that no man is more important than you are to Him. He "is not a man that He should lie" (Numbers 23:19 NKJV), and He says, "I am watching over my word to perform it" (Jeremiah 1:12 ESV). So, the promises of God are for every person who believes and acts on that belief as God directs — even if you don't feel worthy, even if you don't think you qualify. There are some promises, particularly Old Testament promises, that have prerequisites. Jesus fulfilled those prerequisites for us. And more good news — we were redeemed from the curse of the law but not from the blessings! Believe Jesus is who He says He is and did what the Bible tells us He did. That makes every good thing yours.

One last thing about God's being no respecter of persons:

> but if you show partiality, you commit sin...
> - James 2:9 NKJV

I think we all know that God does not sin.

4. We don't rightly divide and discern.

We're Redeemed from the Curse — Not from the Blessings!

You must always keep in mind which covenant the words you read in the Bible are written under. It makes a huge difference in how to receive what's being said. We tend to go the simplest route, dividing between Old Testament and New Testament. But that's not an accurate way to judge. For example, in the Old Testament, Abraham was under an unconditional covenant where all the responsibility was God's, as were the Israelites until the Law was given at Mt. Sinai. Jesus fulfilled ALL conditions, so we get both the Old and New Covenant Promises! The major Biblical covenants are Adamic, Noahic, Abrahamic, Mosaic (the Law), and the New Covenant. There's something to be learned by studying each one. We're not going to go into

Why Don't We Take God's Word at Face Value? | 53

all of these in this book. Just know that we are promised, as grafted in adopted sons, to be recipients of the MANY blessings of the Abrahamic covenant.

> It shall greatly help ye to understand the Scriptures if thou mark not only what is spoken or written, but of whom and to whom, with what words, at what time, where, to what intent, with what circumstances, considering what goeth before and what followeth after.
> - Miles Coverdale 1488-1569
> Bible translator
> Bishop of Exeter

An example of why discernment is important is that Paul often addressed multiple people groups in any given epistle — the new believers, Jews not yet converted, the Gnostics, a certain individual, and whole congregations of the early church. All kinds of doctrinal errors have arisen, due to blanket application of scripture without discernment. For example, what a writer says to a Gnostic regarding the forgiveness of sin is very different from what he'd say to a believer already forgiven. One helpful clue: **Paul addressed only Christians, not even Jews, as *brethren*.** (He knew the value of a clean break.)

You could include considering the historical and cultural context as part of discernment, too. Look at how Jesus answered the Canaanite woman whose daughter was possessed. He called her a dog. How *Christ-like* does that sound? It sounds rude to us today, until we're able to put it in historical context. Jews were special and they knew it. They routinely called Gentiles dogs as an established but derogatory label. Jesus, however, used a gentler term — *kynarion* in Greek, *puppy*, which was used affectionately for pets. In doing so, He softened the term but still tested her resolve. She worshipped Him and made her case for Jesus to deliver her daughter from demons, demonstrating her faith in His power and goodness. So He granted her request even though the time had not yet come for His salvation to be made available to the Gentile nations.

And of course, camels passing through the eye of a needle as an example of the difficulty for a rich man to enter the Kingdom of God is a classic example of our ignorance of historical context. How many people have missed out on the gospel due to that one? The Eye of the Needle was the name of a low arched entrance into a marketplace. As a vendor, if you wanted your camel to carry your goods in, you had to get him on his knees and have him crawl through — not impossible, but difficult. Instead, most people had to unload their goods and carry them in by hand. So a rich man, depicted as often proud of their self-effort, has to humble himself (go down on his knees in humility) to enter the Kingdom.

When questions arise, just take them to God. He loves your questions! Asking questions doesn't mean you don't have faith. He wants to teach you and reveal things to you. When you pursue discernment, the Holy Spirit will provide it. This discernment will finally make sense of those nagging issues that make people think the Bible contradicts itself. I assure you it does not.

Knowing Context and Culture Makes the Bible More Interesting and More Applicable

CHAPTER 7
Settling God's Word

We're now adjusting the lens we look at scripture through, so let's do some fine tuning. We've already found all the promises and all the proof we need that God wants us healed — in the Bible's description of the finished work of the cross, and the definitions of zoe and sozo. It's been there in the Bible all along. Yet many people have already heard it and are still not fully convinced. Not to worry, there are many more proofs.

If you know anything about peoples' names in the Bible and in the Kingdom of God, you know they carry meaning and purpose (example: God changing Abram's name to Abraham, meaning Father of Many Nations). They describe the person's destiny, identity, nature or character. God's names are eternal and are revelatory. They are part of His word to us, so He watches over them to perform them. They are precious to Him because they described to the Israelites, and to everyone who has come after them, Who He is and what He wants to be to us. Here are just a few.

Jehovah Elyon, the Lord Most High
Jehovah Gibbor, the Mighty Lord
Jehovah Tsidkenu, our righteousness
Jehovah Jireh, your provider
Jehovah Raah, your shepherd
Jehovah Nissi, your banner (His banner over me is love.)
Jehovah Shalom, your peace in every circumstance
Jehovah Hoseenu, our maker
Jehovah Shammah, the ever-present
Jehovah Rapha, your healer
Elohim (The God of Israel in plural form, representing Father, Son and Holy Spirit)
El Shaddai (the Almighty, All-Sufficient One)
Yahweh (Lord)
El Roi (the God Who sees you)
Adonai (My great Lord)

There are at least a hundred in all, and they all tell of God's majesty, goodness, love, provision and protection toward you. Meditating on the names of God will reveal what God wants to do and be in your life.

I really need to drive this point home — these names aren't just labels, they're not just descriptions. They ARE. God doesn't just provide; He isn't just the God that provides FOR you. He IS your Provision. He doesn't just heal you; He IS Healing the same way He IS Love and He IS Good.

So names are a really big deal in the Kingdom of God. Nothing carries more power, more importance, more authority, except... Did you know that God placed His Word in a higher place of importance than even His Name?

> I will worship toward thy holy temple, and praise thy name for thy loving kindness and for thy truth: for thou hast magnified thy word above all thy name. - Psalm 138:2 KJV

That's amazing! God placed His Word even above His name! And something else to absorb: Jesus is the Word. God's Word took on flesh and literally became Jesus. How? I have no idea. All I know is that God is God, and there's no better reason to know and love the scriptures than because Jesus IS the Word.

With all this in mind, we'd be wise to elevate the importance we place on the scriptures in our personal lives, don't you think? God's word is settled in heaven (Psalm 119). Nobody debates God's word in heaven, nobody interprets it, nobody picks and chooses which parts they think are true and applicable today. Note that in heaven there is no sin, no sorrow, no sickness, no death. Maybe there's a connection.

> **Confess This Aloud: God Tells the Truth, and I Will Not Doubt What He Says. (Repeat)**

I've said this before — if you want the Word to work in your life, you have to settle in your heart that the Word means what it says, says what it means, and that it's true for YOU. It needs to be as settled in your soul as it is in heaven. Make the Bible your go-to for all truth, and it will repay you hundreds of times over. Remember the scriptures that tell us that God cannot lie? There are several practical reasons this is true.

- The foundation of His throne is justice and righteousness (Psalm 89:14), so if He lied, His throne (rule, sovereignty) would crumble.
- He is watching over His word to perform it. (Jeremiah 1:12)
- If He says it, He is bound by it.
- Whatever He speaks comes into existence, so He literally CANNOT lie.

Hebrews 1:3 in the AMPC says, "He is the perfect imprint and very image of (God's) nature, upholding and maintaining and guiding and propelling the universe by His mighty word of power." The fact that our world hasn't exploded is proof that God's Word works! He chose His words precisely, so you can have confidence that they are true. When you get to the point where there's no room for doubt about the veracity of the scriptures, your life will become an exhibition of God's goodness, and that light will draw others to Him.

> But I the LORD will speak what I will, and it shall be fulfilled without delay... - Ezekiel 12:25 NIV

Every Word God Utters Is a Promise He Will Keep

A Word from our Sponsor: You're wise to rely on God's written word for instruction and for correction in how you approach the subject of healing or any subject. His written word is the Lord's primary method of speaking to us today. But I want you to realize, too, that in the Garden of Eden, there was no Bible. God's original intent was to commune with us, to have direct dialogue with us. That connection is there for you if you'll take advantage of it. Your phone can ring all day, but you won't be able to communicate with the caller if you don't pick it up. You can speak with God constantly, and He'll share wisdom for every situation you find yourself in if you develop your relationship with Him to that extent. Remember the scripture, "If we draw nigh unto Him, He will draw nigh unto us" (James 4:8)? Your relationship with God is up to you. He's waiting. He wants to communicate to you over and above what the Bible tells you — rhema words specific to any given moment. These words will never contradict the Bible, so you can verify them through scripture. Join me in leaning in to Him and deepening the intimacy of our relationships with Him. Meanwhile, every word of the Bible speaks Truth into our circumstances.

Now, back to our scheduled program:

There are countless books in the academic world detailing the proofs of the Bible's authenticity. There are more on its historical accuracy. The ones I'm thinking of right now were written by an unbelieving investigative journalist, a renowned cold case detective, and a university student determined to prove Christianity a lot of hogwash. All three were convinced the Bible was the contrivance of men, and then every one of them got saved due to their own research. All three came to the undeniable conclusion that the Bible is the Word of God and it's true. Why don't those of us who are already saved come to the same conclusion?

There's so much about healing in the Bible that there's just no way, once the veil is off our eyes, to conclude anything other than that God's will is for you to be in peak health all the time. Derek Prince (1915-2003), a pastor in London and best known as a missionary to Africa, had, as a young man in the British Army in Africa, a skin condition that kept him hospitalized for a year. He decided to read the entire Bible and underline every verse pertaining to healing with the blue fountain pen he had there by his hospital bed. I heard him say in an interview, "Do you know what I had when I finished? A blue Bible."

Seeing Isn't Always Believing

You've read about a few of the healings and miracles that have taken place in my life and my person, and some amazing scriptures that tell you healing was provided for everyone.

It's a strange phenomenon, though, that for many, seeing isn't believing, nor is hearing, or reading. We often think, "Well, that's fine for you, but I asked for healing once and it didn't work, so I guess it's just not God's will to heal me," or some other reasoning that's robbing you of your abundant life. Past disappointment, guilt, oratory from a pulpit, your parent's or spouse's opinion, the fact that Aunt Sally (who loved the Lord) died — there are many reasons we don't expect to be healed, if we even dare to hope for it. Again, we must first and foremost believe God's words especially when they contradict what our five senses are telling us. More on that later. But when a person is witness to an obvious example of instantaneous divine healing, you'd expect them to leap into God's arms, right?

One of my dad's best friends (who is also my friend — let's call him Jack) is a genius. He has a very scientific mind. Jack has created many inventions, some of which NASA scientists tested and have not been able to explain the efficiency of. I say this to emphasize his extraordinary intellect, paired with out-of-the-box thinking and a proof-is-in-the-pudding mindset. So his resistance to what he saw with his own eyes is a bit curious.

In early adulthood, Jack oversaw the printing department at his local newspaper. The objective was to keep the presses running. They produced not only the newspaper, but took printing jobs from outside sources.

Every few months a healing evangelist would come through town on his circuit and contract with Jack's office to print the flyers advertising his meetings. This particular early morning, when the evangelist came in to pick up his order, it wasn't ready. Jack and his crew had been working all night. The press had broken down, and while they'd just finished making the repairs, they'd not yet been able to print the flyers. They started the job right away without cleaning up, and the safety covers had not yet been reinstalled on the machinery.

The evangelist, whom I met years later, had his two-year-old daughter with him that morning. As the personnel got the printing job going, Jack and the evangelist stood by chatting. To the best of my memory, here's the way Jack told me about the incident:

"So we're standing there talking over the noise of the presses. He's holding his little girl, and she's squirming because he can't put her down and let her run around. Before we realized what was happening, she leaned over and stuck her hand right in the press! She just stuck her hand right in there! Her scream was terrifying. There was blood everywhere. But the preacher just took her little hand in his and drew it toward his chest, calm as could be, and bowed his head. When he raised it and let go of her hand, it was perfect — not a mark on it, no blood, every joint working. There was still blood all over the presses and the floor, but she wasn't even crying."

Mended by supernatural stitching. Can you imagine witnessing that? Wow — what that would do to your faith, right? Wrong. Yes, this is a great example of a wound being instantly healed through faith, but it's just as good an example of how blind we can allow ourselves to be. It still took thirty years for Jack to come to Christ. Are you allowing yourself to be blind to what Jesus wants to do for you?

Believe the Word Even When It Contradicts Your 5 Senses

Yes, Jack saw the miraculous with his own eyes and still doubted. Even Doubting Thomas believed when he saw. But, there's another lesson on the flip side of this story. We are called to believe not what our eyes see, but what the Word of God says.

Jesus said to him, "Have you believed because you have seen me? Blessed are those who have not seen and yet have believed." - John 20:29 ESV

You are blessed when you know that you were healed two thousand years ago, no matter that you're in pain, no matter what the doctor says, no matter what the lab tech says. You were healed. When you stand on the Word, it WILL come to pass. It accomplishes what God sent it to do. It prosperously affects you. But if you have not settled God's word in your mind and heart, you may not even believe miraculous healings that you see with your own eyes.

> If we accept [as we do] the testimony of men [that is, if we are willing to take the sworn statements of fallible humans as evidence], the testimony of God is greater [far more authoritative]; for this is the testimony of God, that He has testified regarding His Son. - 1 John 5:9 AMP

The Proof is Relationship

God created us to fellowship with Him. But, how can we be in intimate fellowship with somebody whose character we constantly misconstrue? We have so many misconceptions about His will for us as stated in scripture that it's obvious His character is not taught properly in the church overall. When an angry God is taught rather than the Father's love for us through Jesus, then it's no wonder people are waiting for God to launch lightning bolts at them. It's no wonder some of us think illness is our own personal retribution missile launched from heaven. When every insurance policy states that natural disasters are acts of God, how can we think otherwise? When beloved preachers tell us that terrorist attacks, school shootings and plagues are God's punishment for our forsaking Him, how could we know differently? We can get our noses in the Bible, that's how!

I'm going to camp here for a few minutes, if you don't mind. So many people have a shallow, if any, relationship with God because somewhere along the line they've been taught to fear God. Not the reverence and awe of the Biblical word *fear*, but a deep belief that God is angry with them for sins they've committed, that He's watching and waiting for them to step out of line again, and that one day He's going to squash them like a bug through calamity or disease. Nothing could be farther from the truth. Even under the Old Covenant, God promised His people mercy, not wrath. I had a list of about a dozen Old Testament scriptures for you, and that was only a sampling of what God said back then, but decided you might appreciate my just giving you a few I think are the cream.

> "In the time of Noah I promised never again to flood the earth. Now I promise not to be angry with you again; **I will not reprimand or punish you.** - Isaiah 54:9 GNB

If that doesn't reassure you that God's not withholding any good thing from you, I don't know what will.

> Who is a God like you, forgiving iniquity and passing over rebellion for the remnant of his inheritance? He does not hold on to his anger forever because he delights in faithful love. - Micah 7:18 CSB

> And in that day you will say: "O LORD, I will praise You; Though You were angry with me, Your anger is turned away, and You comfort me. - Isaiah 12:1 NKJV

> … For I am God and not man, the Holy One in your midst, And I will not come in wrath… I will heal their apostasy, I will love them freely, For My anger has turned away from them. - Hosea 11:9 NASB & 14:4 ESV

(See how I snuck an extra one in there so it wouldn't seem like so many scriptures to read? Pretty smart, right?)

These are just a few of the many scriptures through which God tells you that He's not angry at you. How many times do you need to hear it? In the New Testament, wrath is mentioned much less often, and then usually as something no longer in effect where believers are concerned:

> For God has not destined us for wrath, but to obtain salvation through our Lord Jesus Christ
> - 1 Thessalonians 5:9 ESV

> Much more then, being now justified by his blood, we shall be saved from wrath through him. - Romans 5:9 KJV

Notice the two New Testament scriptures are both chapter 5, verse 9. Five represents grace. It symbolizes God's lovingkindness and favor to humankind. Nine is a symbol of completeness and finality. Can He make it any more obvious? His work is complete, and grace is his final word to you. You are not destined for wrath — quite the opposite.

When you examine God's character in the Word, even just by reading the list of His Names at the beginning of this chapter, you can't help but realize that He's not punishing you and He wants **only** the best of everything for you. Remember, Jesus is the flesh and blood manifestation of the nature of the Father and of His Word.

Question: Who were the only ones Jesus chastised? Answer: Hypocritical, unbelieving religious leaders. He was never angry with the thieves, prostitutes or social outcasts. They were the ones he had compassion for.

Like many of us, Adam and Eve were afraid and hid from God after they sinned; whereas, before their disobedience, they had looked forward to their daily walk with Him in the garden. Note that God didn't rebuke Adam and Eve; He called them to Him. He didn't chastise them; He clothed them. He didn't send them into darkness; He killed animals to serve as sacrifices in their stead. He did not punish them by throwing them out of the garden; He protected them from living eternally on this earth in that sin state by barring the way to the Tree of Life. Everything He did then, and everything Jesus did four thousand years later, was to restore the relationship between Man and God — your Father God — whose nature is revealed in His Names.

In fellowshipping with Him, let Him reveal His truth and love to you. If you've ever feared God's wrath, you're going to find a very different God than you've expected in the past.

Relationships are powerful forces in our lives. Years ago, our church organized us into cell groups. The pastors determined how many groups were needed to include everyone in the congregation and enlisted that many couples within the church to serve as group leaders/hosts. We were to meet in their homes one night each week, eat together, and participate in a study or further discuss the sermon we'd heard at church a few days earlier. Most importantly, we were to build relationships and support each other in whatever life threw at us. The sign-up sheets were in the lobby, with a local map showing the location of each host home so that we could determine our closest group geographically. By the time Kevin and I made it to the lobby, the closest group to our home was filled.

Kevin said, "Hey, let's join THIS one — Kathy and Randall's. It's not too far away."

"No! Not that one. See, here. This one's closer."

"Not really. I think this is the one."

"No, honey, I don't want to join that one. Pick another."

"Why? What's wrong with..."

And on it went until we were officially signed up for the Battenburg's group. Three days of misery— that was the countdown to the first cell group meeting. What was my problem? Intimidation. Kathy was a tall, willowy beauty. They'd started attending about the same time as us, but Kathy was regularly asked to sing, and when she did, she had carte blanche to say whatever she felt led to say from the pulpit. And she was eloquent, on and off stage. She was a professional woman and also sang and ministered in very impressive venues outside of our church. She was all the things I'd thought at a younger age I'd be. But my life had taken different twists and turns, so I'd not pursued things that engendered or required those talents and abilities. Not only had I not achieved those things, I felt I'd lost some of them. I was tongue-tied around her. When I saw her, I looked for a detour to avoid contact. I was deeply intimidated because I felt deeply inferior. When my husband finally got me to admit the problem, he thought I was being ridiculous, but that didn't change how I felt.

Their home was welcoming; everyone was open and warm. Kathy spoke freely about what was going on in their life, and when she told a very funny, very southern story of something that had recently happened, every ounce of my intimidation melted away. The moment she became personal to me was the moment my intimidation fled, and I began to just love her. I felt like I was with family.

A few months later, I admitted to her that I'd been intimidated by her, and do you know what her response was? She laughed. Not a politely amused laugh, I'm talking a could-barely-catch-her-breath belly laugh! By then we had become the best of friends, speaking on the phone most days, our families going out to lunch after church regularly, dropping in on each other, supporting each other through difficult times — doing what friends do. Now, many years later, though we're thousands of miles apart, when we're together in person or on the phone, it's almost as if we've never been separated.

Remember I said I felt I was with family? Kathy and her husband came to my dad's funeral. She looks so much like my own kin that a family member actually asked me, "Which cousin is that? I can't quite place her." She's the younger image of my wonderful Aunt Susan, one of my favorite people in the whole world, even having similarities in career and personality. Yet, I had thought her unapproachable.

The devil is a liar.

Is the enemy lying to you about God's approachability? In what state is your relationship with Him? How approachable do you feel He is? Do you KNOW that He loves you and wants you well even more than you want you well? Can you spontaneously enter the throne room — just stop whatever you're doing and thinking and begin to praise and worship Him from deep in your spirit? How do you pray? Do you think about what you're going to say to Him so it sounds like your pastor's praying from the pulpit, or do you just talk to Him like He's your Dad? Are you intimidated by Him, or do you seek His presence throughout the day?

We are so inferior to God, yet He longs for an intimate relationship with each of us, His crowning achievements. He is infinite, so each one of us can have His undivided attention 24/7. Did you know you are His favorite child? Do you act like you know it? He wants you to desire to spend time with Him, to have the kind of relationship where you can feel comfortable and be yourself. He created you that way, and He longs to spend time with the one He created. You're His masterpiece.

Good Relationships Are Gifts from God – A Good Relationship WITH God is Up to You

Unless you have a personal relationship with God, you won't sincerely believe the wonders of the scriptures because they're too good to be true in the natural. You have to get to know Him, in order to believe He could be that good. NOW is the time to deepen your relationship with the personages of your God. NOW is the time to become closer, transparent (He knows, anyway) and unceasing in prayer. The closer you are to God, the easier it is for Him to reveal His truth to you. The closer you are to God, the more aware you are of how great His love is toward you and the easier it is to receive. The closer you are to God the easier it is to hear His strategies and instructions that will lead you out of every difficulty, including illness.

Pursue Him for Who He is, not for what He can do for you, "and all these things shall be added unto you" (Matthew 6:33).

Developing a relationship is much easier when you're well than when you're in a crisis, but it's never too late. Pursue Him NOW, regardless of the condition of your body at this time. You don't have a minute to lose.

CHAPTER 8
Wash Your Brain

Renewing your mind isn't about how much scripture you know. There are many people who can spout the King James word for word, but do life looking like they were weaned on lemons. It's about how much of God's light you've allowed to penetrate your mind. Atheists and science-y types would agree that where there is a lack of knowledge, darkness prevails. This statement is particularly true when referring to a lack of knowledge of God. (He IS all knowledge, after all.) Knowledge of God, knowing His character, His love, your identity in Christ, His plan for your life — all of this shines a light in your darkness, and where there is light, darkness cannot prevail.

Proverbs 3:5 cautions us not to rely on our own understanding. Guard against believing something just because it's what you want to be true, because it's what you've always been told or because it makes sense to you. We so easily believe lies. Decide to believe only what God believes. Anything short of that is detrimental.

Another tendency we humans have is to decide for ourselves who, what, or how God is. That is setting yourself up as God! He is almighty — you are not, I am not. He is Who He says He is, not who we say He is. It is our privilege to search Him out, pursue Him, and enter into relationship with Him. But we do not get to bend Him into what we want Him to be. To believe He is other than Whom He reveals Himself to be through His Word is to jeopardize your eternity. Discovering His true nature and character is both the process and the product of renewing your mind.

Believing correctly on any particular subject can come instantly — a flash of revelatory understanding, and your mindset is forever changed. Most times, though, you have to pursue correct beliefs — track them down, capture them, consume them. It is vital to read the scriptures with your spiritual eyes open and with the help of the Holy Spirit. Begin right now to deepen your personal relationship with God, no matter what stage it's in at this moment. Pursue Him through examining His Word and fellowshipping with Him.

Abandoning long-held beliefs is so hard. I understand — I've been there and sometimes find

> Questioning Long-Held Beliefs Is Difficult – but the Pay-Off Can Be Huge

myself right back there. I would say that renewing your mind is probably most difficult when you feel you are already close to God and know His Word. You think that if you were believing wrongly for the last twenty years, He would have told you so by now. But God's access to our hearts and minds can be limited by what we already believe, and by our egos and stubbornness in thinking we already know. He doesn't love us any less because of it, but we're still missing out on God's best for us. We're still wrong. When we hear that still, small voice talking to us about certain subjects, we tell ourselves it's the enemy trying to deceive us. Sometimes, it's the voice of God we're refusing to recognize because we "know" what we just heard couldn't possibly be true. You're right — it couldn't be true…unless some of the stuff you already believe is wrong. Ask the Holy Spirit to remove the veil from your eyes and ears, and you'll be able to confirm that voice by scripture, thereby renewing your mind as commanded. You can always learn more about an infinite being. It's worth the effort — this is a chance to get to know God better. Don't be afraid — He will confirm His truth to you.

I was thirty when I finally had an opportunity to learn scuba diving. Immediately, I wished I had taken lessons when I was sixteen, because I'd now lived twice as long, cementing in my mind the *fact* that humans cannot breathe underwater. I had to renew my mind to the idea of swimming without surfacing for air. Once I broke through that belief system, I could enjoy the amazing new world before me. That breakthrough didn't only have to happen once, though. I had to overcome that mindset many times as I rolled backwards off the side of a boat, but each time became easier. Eventually, I didn't have to think about it anymore.

What happens is that we never move beyond that first revelation of God. The church we got saved in tends to dictate the box we keep God in our whole lives. Why is that? Faith comes by hearing, and that's what we heard, true or not, complete or not. Break free! Be a Christ-follower, not a religion devotee. Understand, I really don't care whether you're sprinkled or dunked. The danger is in the teachings that deny what God plainly states. Some denominational congregations let God reign, and I applaud them. Non-denominationalism might be a good step in a general sense, but it's not always enough. Churches that call themselves non-denominational are often just a repackaged version of whatever denomination the leadership came out of, less the accountability. Regardless of what banner your church puts itself under, if they restrict God or restrain you from believing what the Bible states in plain English, Greek, and Hebrew, then find a different church. Besides, the united church that Jesus will return for is not going to be labeled by any name but His.

> And be not conformed to this world, but be ye transformed by the renewing of your mind, that ye may prove what [is] that good, and acceptable, and perfect, will of God.
> - Romans 12:2 KJV

Denomination and Denominator Come from the Same Root Word — They Both Divide

This is probably the best-known scripture pertaining to renewing your mind. I looked up several words in the Greek, and unpacking this verse, we see that mind renewal (*Strong's* G342 - *anakainosis* - *def. renovate, complete change for the better*), in this case by the Word of God, transforms you from the inside out. It changes your belief system to conform with God's. But you have to be willing for the veil over your spiritual eyes to be removed. As you are transformed, you are able to prove (*Strong's* G1381 - *dokimazo* - *def.* "discern, recognize as genuine after examination") what the will of God is. The more of the Word you get into you, the more you will be able to understand God's will.

> For to be carnally minded is death, but to be spiritually minded is life and peace. - Romans 8:6 KJV

> For as he thinks in his heart, so is he. - Proverbs 23:7 KJV

What You Believe Becomes What You Say; What You Say Becomes What You Have

And as that living, powerful Word transforms you, your thoughts begin to line up with God's thoughts. As your thought life improves, you'll see positive changes in other areas. Your thoughts are seeds that bear fruit in your life!

> "Throw off all the transgressions you have committed, and get yourselves a new heart and a new spirit. Why should you die, house of Israel? For I take no pleasure in anyone's **death**." This is the declaration of the Lord God. "So repent and **live**!" - Ezekiel 18:31,32 CSB

In Chapter 6 we searched out the meaning of the Hebrew words maveth (*death, dying, state of death*) and chaya (*live, remain alive, live prosperously, revive from sickness, discouragement or death*). Those are the words used here in Ezekiel 18:32. This passage explains to us that God is not happy about ANYONE's death, and if we change our minds around what we think God's intentions are pertaining to our physical bodies, we will live.

In other words, renew your mind so that you will not die!

Scripture as Medicine

> My son, give attention to my words; Incline your ear to my sayings. Do not let them depart from your eyes; Keep them in the midst of your heart. For they are life to those who find them, And **health to all their flesh**.
> - Proverbs 4:20-22 NKJV

Health to all their flesh — what does that mean? It means exactly what it says. It's pretty difficult to spiritualize the word *flesh*. The CSB translates it, "for they are life to those who find them and health to one's whole body." That's pretty clear. **The Word will save your life. It will make you healthy. It will heal you.** God's Word (Jesus) IS health. God is YOUR health.

The day my husband and I finally learned to take scriptures into us as if they were medicine was the day he learned healing was really possible. He was in Korea, and we later discovered, bleeding internally. He was so weak he could hardly put one foot in front of the other. Being oceans away, I could only judge his condition based on his voice. It went from not much more than a whisper even after a night's sleep, to sounding vital and strong even after a hectic day's work. Within three days of learning to take the Word as medicine, he was a different person!

Use scripture as medicine. You can take that as literally as you like. Choose some healing scriptures and write them on index cards. Then, every three or four hours, just as you would for medication, read them aloud to yourself. Set a timer if needed to remind yourself to take the next "dose". Meditate on those verses as you go about your day. It's very effective. I have a friend that printed out Keith Moore's list of personalized scriptures (available on his website), and she reads the entire list of a hundred verses aloud every day to stay healthy. It's amazing how no matter how many times she reads them a particular scripture will on different days just arrest her, and God will show her something amazing in that verse she hasn't seen before. The Word is alive and powerful. It brings life wherever it is planted, so sow it into your body!

> Facts Change in the Face of Truth

What's the most important thing to know about taking God's Word as medicine? That God's Word is true, of course. Remember this one?

> God is not a man, that He should lie, or a son of man, that he should change his mind. Has he said, and will he not do it? Or has he spoken and will he not fulfill it? Behold, I have received a command to bless; he has blessed and I cannot revoke it. - Numbers 23:19,20 ESV

By the way, if you are using prescription drugs, bless them before you take them, and stand on the scripture that nothing poisonous can harm you. (I do this with food, too, as it's often so unhealthy these days.)

The Father's Desire

Paul says healing is elementary. It's foundational. He healed people every day. When he and the disciples crossed paths with a person who needed healing, they healed him. Not believing in healing is so far from the gospel that Paul really never addressed unbelief in that area. Here's how he expressed the part healing plays in the gospel:

> ...leaving the discussion of the ELEMENTARY PRINCIPLES of Christ, let us go on to perfections, Not laying again the FOUNDATION of repentance from dead works and faith toward God, of the doctrine of baptisms, of LAYING ON OF HANDS, of resurrection of the dead, and of eternal judgement. - Hebrews 6:1,2 NKJV

He was saying, let's get to some meat, and stop all this discussion of milk — surely, you're ready for some meat by now. Yet here we are, two thousand years later, still debating whether divine healing is for today. I hate to say it, but the devil has done a bang-up job of convincing the church that God wants us sick and in lack. What do you want for your children? I bet it's not for them to be sick.

James was writing to brand new believers, and he said, "IF there are any sick among you..." In other words, there shouldn't be, but if any of you are still sick even though you got saved, then call the elders and they'll deal with that, because it shouldn't be an issue in your life now that you're a Christian. The early church left no room for sickness. The only ailments they suffered came about through persecution.

> **Faith Isn't Believing God Can, It's Knowing He Already Has**

Healing is the biggest draw even today that God has to offer, in the minds of the pre-saved. It's the number one reason people seek God out — because most everyone wants to live. And if it's the biggest draw of people toward God, then it's what the enemy most wants to undermine.

> ...and a great multitude of the people... came to hear him, and to be healed of their sicknesses, and those harassed by unclean spirits, and they were healed, and all the multitude were seeking to touch him, because power from him was going forth, and he was healing all. - Luke 6:17-19 YLT

They came! People are drawn to healing like flies to honey. That's why so much confusion and dissention exists around healing. Our enemy, being the liar and deceiver he is, knows that if he creates confusion and doubt and acrimony around healing, the body of Christ (the church) will remain sick and powerless. Not only that, but we won't be able to minister healing to the lost world, resulting in fewer people coming to Christ.

Well that's all changing, folks, because our Father God is calling the world to Him now more than ever, as the return of Christ draws closer each and every day. He would love for every Christian on the planet to be affirming the gospel out in the streets, at their jobs, at the grocery store, in every aspect of their daily lives, by healing every sick person they encounter, and bringing in new believers daily – acting like the early church.

What does the Bible say? Whatever it says is what God wants for you. It's settled. So, are you ready to see how closely your beliefs about healing line up with God's Word? Remember, the Word reveals His will, and we're supposed to be enforcing His will here and now. Let's pray before we examine the doctrines we've lived by for so long.

Father God, I open my heart to you right now. I want to receive Your truth and only Your truth. I submit myself to receive from You. Holy Spirit, open my eyes to see, renew my mind, and place your Truth deep in my soul so that I can apply it in my life. Pull back the veil so that I understand what you are saying to ME in the Word. I want everything you have for me, Lord, and I recognize that you will not give me a stone when I ask for bread. You created Truth, and I ask You to reveal it to me today. You instigated all spiritual laws. Show me, Lord, how they are to operate in my life. Because I am Your child I have everything necessary for life and godliness here on this earth. Teach me, Lord, how to draw those things out from your Spirit living inside me and from your Word and apply them now in my everyday life. Amen.

Part Four
DEADLY DOCTRINES: MAN'S WISDOM, THE ENEMY'S LIES

He answered them, "And why do you break the commandment of God for the sake of your tradition?"
- Matthew 15:3 ESV

He (Jesus) answered them, "Isaiah prophesied correctly about you hypocrites, as it is written: This people honors me with their lips, but their heart is far from me." They worship me in vain, teaching as doctrines human commands. Abandoning the command of God, you hold on to human tradition." - Mark 7: 6-13 CSB

And be renewed in the spirit of your mind;
- Ephesians 4:23 KJV

And be not conformed to this world, but be ye transformed by the renewing of your mind, that ye may prove what [is] that good, and acceptable, and perfect, will of God.
- Romans 12:2 KJV

CHAPTER 9
Holding on to Human Traditions

> And it came to pass on a certain day, as he was teaching, that there were Pharisees and doctors of the law sitting by, which were come out of every town of Galilee, and Judaea, and Jerusalem: and the power of the Lord was present to heal them. - Luke 5:17 KJV

In the original writing, the word *present* was not included; that was added through man's wisdom. Man's way of *improving* this scripture makes it sound as if sometimes the power is there, sometimes it's not. But "The power of the Lord was to heal them," reveals God's nature. This was the day a paralyzed man was lowered through the roof by his friends for Jesus to heal him. Did other people get healed that day? Of course, that's how Jesus rolls. Did any Pharisees get healed? I think a miracle that momentous would have been mentioned. The Pharisees wanted nothing from Jesus except his death. But this scripture in its original form makes it clear that healing was available to them and even that God desired to heal them, although their hearts were darkened toward his son.

We've established by the scriptural accounts that when Jesus walked this earth, He healed every infirm person He encountered — because it was the Father's will, and He was empowered by the Holy Spirit. We have scriptural proof that Jesus is alive and that He doesn't need to be present to heal. We have scriptural proof that all believers can now walk in power with the Holy Spirit. We have scriptural proof that God's character never changes and that He cannot lie. Therefore, His promises are true, and His will for His children cannot change.

Yet we've seen so many people disappointed, and so many people die, that we don't truly believe He heals today.

But we still pray for it.

We pray faithless prayers for healing, or at least for the abatement of symptoms or the strength to endure them. In other words, most of us don't want to be ill, but we hedge our bets by praying, "...if it be Thy will" because we don't really expect results from our prayers, and we aren't the least bit certain God really wants to heal us. And then, if we're hoping against hope that we just might get healed but aren't healed soon enough to suit us, we make excuses for God — "He's teaching me humility, or patience, or penitence," or "He's going to get the glory for this. My suffering is going to inspire so many!" What little faith you had, you just flushed.

The Only Person Who Can Defeat God's Promises in Your Life Is YOU

Most of us, in the deepest shadows of our intellect, believe we're not healed because we're being punished for those deep, dark sins. You know, the ones you try not to remember — the ones you can't admit to anyone because you're afraid, and sometimes rightly so, that you'll lose your friends and be cast out of your church.

Then there's the ever-popular thorn in Paul's side. Surely that's proof that God makes you sick, or at least allows sickness, for His own purposes. Right?

Many believe miracles could only be performed when the Apostles lived, and therefore, healing now only manifests when you get to heaven. They say, "Even those that Jesus raised from the dead eventually died again, so there's no such thing as real healing here in this life." Some even feel God is calling them home when they get sick.

We're going to look at these and other prevalent belief structures regarding healing that exist within the church today to see how they line up with what God says through His Word. After all, **God's is the only opinion that matters**. His is Truth. But, believe it or not, you can defeat the power of God's truth in your own life and, unfortunately, in the lives of those you influence. I'm going to repeat that because it is incredibly important: God's Word, His will for your life will not be borne out if you don't believe it, and you can be responsible for holding back your children and others you have influence over by your words and example when your beliefs don't line up with what God says.

> For you will no longer remember the oracle of the Lord, because every man's own word will become the oracle; and you have perverted the words of the living God, the Lord of Hosts, our God. - Jeremiah 23:36 AMP

> That your faith should not stand in the wisdom of men, but in the power of God. - 1 Corinthians 2:5 KJV

So by this you have invalidated the word of God (depriving it of force and authority and making it of no effect) for the sake of your tradition (handed down by the elders). You hypocrites (play-actors, pretenders), rightly did Isaiah prophesy of you when he said, "This people honors Me with their lips, but their heart is far away from Me. But in vain do they worship Me, for they teach as doctrines the precepts of men." - Matthew 15: 6-9 AMP

Unbelief is Adultery Toward God

English dictionaries define *unbelief* as the state or quality of not believing; incredulity or skepticism, especially in matters of doctrine or religious faith. But the Greek word for unbelief, *apistia*, is defined as unfaithful, the same as being unfaithful to your spouse. God sees unbelief as adultery. That is how God described Israel's relationship with Him when they fell into idolatry and unbelief.

>...And anything that is not based on faith is sin.
>- Romans 14:23 GNT

>But the doubter comes under condemnation...because his action is not based on trust. And anything not based on trust is a sin. - Romans 14:23 CJB

Make no mistake; unbelief is sin.
So is DISbelief, which is the REFUSAL to accept something that is true or real. You can walk in unbelief due to ignorance, you can walk in unbelief due to what circumstances you see in the natural world, or you can walk in unbelief due to disbelief — your own refusal to accept God's Truth when you've heard it. So do not be fooled any longer. God's Word is true whether you believe it or not.

Remember that in Mark 16:14, Jesus rebuked the disciples for their "unbelief and hardness of heart" because they did not believe the reports of those who saw Him after He had risen. He rebuked THE DISCIPLES for not believing somebody who was not a disciple. Life lesson: you may think you know more scripture, have studied more theology, or are spiritually ahead of some other Christian, but your *status* is irrelevant to God. Remember, God is no respecter of persons. Sometimes brand-new Christians will blow you away with the extent of their revelation — it stems from the purity of their faith. And sometimes those with the most theological knowledge and training are the ones not living in the love and blessings of God — not thriving, living paycheck to paycheck, catching the illness du jour, living with a chronic condition, or growling at people instead of sharing the love of God. Or you may be doing everything right, saying the right things, serving tirelessly, yet not having that intimate personal relationship because you just don't believe He's as good as He is. Do not trust in what you think you know — make room for God to reveal more to you, even if the source surprises you.

> So we see that because of their unbelief they were not able to enter his rest. - Hebrews 3:19 NLT

There's always more in God. The good news when it comes to unbelief is that God is merciful, and you're already forgiven. It's OK to start with, "I believe Lord! Help Thou my unbelief" (Mark 9:24)! I've quoted that one to Him quite a few times. And He doesn't hold it against you—He rejoices over your acceptance of His truths when that day comes. Even Paul was in that same position:

> ...But I received mercy because I acted out of ignorance in unbelief, and the grace of our Lord overflowed, along with the faith and love that are in Christ Jesus.
> - 1 Timothy 1:13,14 CSB

Faith Comes by Hearing Not Having Heard So Stay in the Word

So if you're walking in unbelief around healing, when God, according to His scriptural promises, wants you healed, why? Every single time you don't believe what God (Who cannot lie) says, it's because you have an erroneous belief in that area. In other words, you have believed a lie — a lie from the enemy — even though it may have been spoken by somebody you trusted, even though it may have come from a pulpit, even though you feel a scripture was disproven by God's failure to heal a loved one in the past. If what you believe right now doesn't line up with the promises in His Word, then you are believing a lie from the pit of hell.

So repent — change your belief! None of us is infallible, and that's why God gave us the Bible — to verify or invalidate what you hear and even experience. It's also why God called me to write this book. I can tell you from experience that it's hard to unlearn years of doctrine, but that's exactly what you must do in order to believe God. If you're new to the family of God, then you'll find renewing your mind to the Word much easier because you're starting fresh. Open mind, insert Truth.

You can ask God a specific question, and He will give you a specific answer in such a way that there is no doubt. Once my pastor mentioned in a sermon the scripture, "Taste and see that the Lord is good" (Psalm 34:8). I told God that it made no sense to me. I could relate to the other senses revealing Him, but how do you taste God? When I went down front for prayer and worship with many others at the end of the service, my mouth suddenly filled with the most incredible flavor. It was better than tree-ripened mangoes in the Philippines. I can't describe it, but I can remember it at will to enjoy it all over again. He will impart truth to you in tangible ways that will settle questions for you once and for all. He won't leave you hanging. When you get an answer directly from God Almighty, no other opinion will hold merit.

But here's the mistake most people make: forgetting that God continues to reveal more and more to you, IF YOU WILL

Precept — A Rule Intended to Regulate Behavior or Thought

RECEIVE IT, regardless of how long you've been a Christian. And He reveals more and more to the church at large as we get closer and closer to Jesus' return. Once you're saved, the rest of your life should include a constant renewing of your mind to the truths of God. You can never know everything about an infinite being. So expect to hear God, and remain ready to hear more. When you ask for bread, He will not give you a stone, but neither will He give you meat when you're still gumming the pablum. There's no condemnation in that. Everyone progresses at different rates in different areas of life and knowledge of Him, according to their own experiences, what they've been taught in the past, what they're listening to now, and what they're trying to get answers for.

Right now, you're want to know if you can receive divine healing. You cannot — not by believing man-made doctrines that are fueled by men's attempts to achieve in their own strength what God offers us freely. Those precepts make God's Word ineffective and powerless if you believe them. But believing the Word means there's no end to what God can do in and through you. So let's see what the Bible says on the subject and debunk some of the lies from satan you may be believing.

9 Head-Smackers that Prove God Wants You Healed

1. The Good Father

How do you feel when your child is ill? You just want to kiss him and make it all better, right? Do you think you're a kinder parent than God? Do you love your children more than God does? More than He loves YOU? Impossible.

Father with a capital F — Abba (Daddy) — is simply the best parent in the universe. Ever. Even if you had a wonderful loving dad, one who never raised his voice and only explained rather than punished, he is evil compared to God, no offence to your dad. But in comparison to God, that is true.

> If you then, who are evil, know how to give good gifts to your children, how much more will your Father who is in heaven give good things to those who ask him!
> - Matthew 7:11 ESV

> See what kind of love the Father has given to us, that we should be called children of God; and so we are…
> - 1 John 3:1 ESV

And for those who believe God **makes** us sick, how could he? Only a warped human could rationalize treating his children that way. God has infinite ways to lead, guide, teach, and direct you without causing you harm. No, that's your enemy the devil making you sick, not your loving Heavenly Father. Pair these two scriptures together.

> How precious, O God, is your **constant love!** We find protection under the **shadow of your wings**.
> - Psalm 26:7 GNT

> But unto you that fear my name shall the Sun of righteousness arise with **healing in his wings** …
> - Malachi 4:2 KJV

His *constant love*…Did you know that the tassels, or the hem, of Jewish prayer shawls is called the "wings"? What was it that the woman with the issue of blood said? "If I can but touch the hem of his garment, I will be healed." God's word is so beautiful. And everything is tied together to give us proof after proof of its truth and His constant love.

Get that picture in your mind, God as He really is, the most loving parent ever to exist in all the universe. Dwell on that for a few minutes, right now. Just take a moment...meditate on the perfect Father.

Now do you think He wants you healed? He absolutely does. Who's your Daddy?

2. Healing as Evangelism

> And He went about doing good and healing ALL who were oppressed by the devil, because God was with Him.
> - Acts 10:38 AMP

BECAUSE *God was with Him* —clearly healing is God's will. Jesus healed all *because God was with Him.*

> Whenever you go into a city and they welcome you, eat what is set before you, and heal those in it who are sick (authenticating your message), and say to them, 'The kingdom of God has come near to you.'
> - Luke 10:8-9 AMP

This scripture refers to when the 70 were sent out ahead of Jesus. They were not instructed to pray to determine who was eligible for healing according to worthiness. He instructed them to heal **everyone** who was sick in **every** city they entered. And note that this was a way of authenticating their message of the Kingdom of God. You cannot see with your eyes when somebody receives forgiveness of their sins, so that is not how the Gospel is authenticated. Healing is. It is proof of God's goodness and proof that the Gospel is true. Healing is the primary tool in God's evangelical toolbox! If He could experience frustration, this would be the time, when healing is right there in front of us and we can't figure out how to access it. Even worse is when there are other people who need healing and saving, and we don't even try to help them because we're believing lies. Paul said:

> And my message and my preaching were not couched in
> specious words of philosophy but were dependent for their
> efficacy upon a demonstration of the SPIRIT and of
> POWER, in order that your FAITH should not be resting
> in human philosophy but IN GOD'S POWER.
> - 1 Corinthians 2:4,5 WET

If **Jesus and Paul** didn't rely on words only, but **on the demonstration of the power of God**, how on earth is it that we think we're supposed to get people saved by our words alone? Does it happen? Sure, by God's grace through faith (Ephesians 2:8). But why would we think God would stop supplying the power to authenticate His gospel? MORE people get saved when they see the power demonstrated, and God still wants everyone saved, doesn't he? He heals because it is His nature. But it is unsaved man's nature to more readily believe when he sees proof.

3. Enter His Gates with Thanksgiving

> ...And I will heal him (making his lips blossom anew with
> thankful praise) - Isaiah 57:19 AMP

What a sweet picture of His goodness drawing you near. The Lord loves to receive our praise almost as much as He loves blessing us. What's more, as with everything God tells us to do, praising Him is for OUR benefit. His blessings are self-perpetuating in a sense because in praising, we are blessed. Praising Him makes us stronger in the spirit. It's nearly identical to encouraging ourselves in the Lord. God once said to Abraham, "Blessing I will bless you." It's brilliant.

4. Victory Over Satan

Acts 10:38, "...healing all who were oppressed by the devil, because God was with Him," tells us not only that healing is God's will, but also that illness is oppression of the devil, the enemy of God! Pretty strong words, but they're not mine. They're God's. Does God still oppose satan? Of course, He does. Therefore, He wants you healed today to foil His enemy's trap that you stumbled into.

> ... so that through His death He might destroy the one
> holding the power of death — that is, the devil...
> - Hebrews 2:14 CSB

5. Supplying the Church

> So God has appointed and placed in the church...those with the gifts of healings... - 1 Corinthians 12:28 AMP

Does the church still exist? Yes, it does. Then you are supposed to have brothers and sisters in Christ who minister the gifts of healings. That would not be the case if healing were not God's will.

6. The Lord's Prayer

We pray as Jesus taught, "Thy will be done on earth as it is in heaven." You know beyond the shadow of a doubt that His will is done in heaven, and Jesus instructs you to ask, even declare, that His will be done here on earth, too. Is there any sickness in heaven? We know from Scripture there is not. So if it's not His will in heaven, are you saying that sickness is His will on earth? It can't be — that would contradict Jesus' instruction on how to pray. Therefore, we're praying at Jesus' instruction and in agreement with the Father's Will, every time we pray the Lord's Prayer, for there to be no sickness on earth. Did you realize that was in the Lord's Prayer?

When we pray, we're supposed to believe that we receive what we've asked for in agreement with His Will (Mark 11:24). Do you? An important note: nothing in this prayer begs God to do anything. Instead, it declares God's will and commands that it manifest here on earth. That's how we're supposed to pray when there's a job to accomplish, because we have dominion.

7. Our Provider

> His divine power has given us everything we need for life (zoe)...- 2 Peter 1:3 BSB

> He who did not spare his own Son, but gave him up for us all — how will he not also, along with Him, graciously give us all things? - Romans 8:32 NIV

This scripture in Romans clearly states that The Father and Jesus will graciously (many translations say "freely") give you all things. Why? He's already given you the greatest gift and blessing possible — eternal life with Him in which there is no sorrow or sickness. Before you were saved, when you were still an enemy of God and had no understanding of His love, Jesus sacrificed Himself for this purpose. So since we who are saved are now His children, why wouldn't He give us these lesser gifts, blessings that cost Him nothing above what He's already given? He watched the brutal suffering and death of His only begotten son for your benefit and mine, so why would you think He wouldn't give you some spare parts, which is all healing is? And He gives it freely — abundantly and at no charge! You don't get a bill, you can't earn it, and you don't have to suffer for it. A blessing is just that — a blessing. If it were possible to work for it, then it wouldn't be a blessing. He would owe it to you, making it about your works, not His grace.

> For if, while we were enemies, we were Reconciled to God through the death of his Son, then how much more, having been reconciled, will we be saved (*sozo*) by his life (zoe).
> - Romans 5:10 CSB

8. God and Medicine

If you don't believe that healing is God's will for you or you believe that God makes you sick or is calling you home, why are you going against his will by going to the doctor to get well? "I believe He's given us doctors for this modern age," you might say. OK then, why would He do that if he doesn't want you healed? So He does want you healed. You just established that. Now, do you want to be healed through surgery and prescription drugs with side effects and spend all your life savings like the woman with the issue of blood, or would you rather be healed instantly, now, by your Heavenly Abba? By all means go to the doctor—at least to have your healing confirmed.

9. Sacrifices

What did God say about our sacrifices to Him? They were to be unblemished. When the Israelites began sacrifices according to God's instructions, the animal was selected, examined outwardly for imperfections — sores, wounds, scars, skin blemishes. Then the priests had to be sure no illness was present, so the lamb was observed for symptoms of disease for three days before being declared acceptable. (Three days, get it?) Jesus, being the perfect lamb of God, was free from all illness and blemishes until His passion began. Now, in New Covenant days, there are no more animal sacrifices. WE are the sacrifices.

I'll be honest. I preach to myself with this whole book, but nowhere more than right here. This is a stunning revelation.

> I urge you therefore, brothers, by the mercies of God, that you present your **bodies** as a living sacrifice, holy, and acceptable to God, which is your reasonable service of worship. - Romans 12:1 MEV

It doesn't say your heart, your mind, your spirit, your soul, your emotions or your intentions, but *your body*. You are the hands and feet of Jesus on this earth. You need to be functional. You are called to present your body every day as a living sacrifice, holy and acceptable to the Lord. Search the scriptures — the rules for the condition of sacrifices have not changed! God has given you power and authority over the enemy. Now you can ensure that as a sacrifice your body is unblemished — whole, healed, able — acceptable. Awesome. This revelation was shared with me by my friend, author Shontesha Price, who rid her body of 23 chronic symptoms, some she'd had her entire life without medical resolution. Use the authority Jesus gives you as His ambassador in this world to make and keep your body healthy — acceptable as an unblemished living sacrifice. Powerful.

CHAPTER 10
Healing is not for Today

Healing Manifests in Heaven

Let's go ahead and get this doctrine out of the way, as so many other misunderstandings are rooted here. After the flood, God put a limit on our physical lives. Unless you're raptured first, your body is going to die at some point. Healing isn't about whether or not you die. **Healing is about when and how you die.**

> And Jesus having uttered a loud cry, yielded the spirit, - Mark 15:37 YLT

> The days of Abraham's life were 175 years. Then Abraham's spirit was released, and he died at a good (ample, full) old age, an old man, satisfied and satiated, and was gathered to his people. - Genesis 25:7-8 AMPC

How should a Christian die? Do you know where the phrase *give up the ghost* came from? The fathers of our faith decided when it was time to join the Lord, and at that time they sat down and released their spirits to Him. Well-known Baptist pastor and author E.W. Kenyon did the same. In fact, that's exactly what my father-in-law did. He decided it was time, and in twenty minutes, he was gone.

There are many examples of modern-day Christians who have done just that. "Well, it's time. I'm ready to go. I love you all, and I'm going to lay down now because I'm going to heaven at 10 a.m. sharp. I'll see you later." I recently heard of a woman in Georgia who died at 111 years old. She decluttered her house first so the *kids* didn't have to deal with it. Then she phoned all the children and grand-children and great-grands and possibly great-great grands and told them she was going home, and if they wanted to see her before she left, it was time to come. When asked what the secret to her longevity was, she replied, "Honey, I don't worry '*bout nuthin!*" Brilliant — peace prolongs life, stress kills.

We read the Bible to find out how God wants us to *do life*. It's all about living our best life here and leading as many as possible into eternity in heaven. Your *best life* does not include sickness and disease.

You don't even take your body with you to heaven, so why would you need healing there? If healing is for after you arrive in heaven, why did Jesus heal here on earth? And how could He? Why didn't He just say, "There's no pain or disease in heaven, so you have that to look forward to if you believe in Me."

And if healing is only for heaven, why are we instructed to go to the elders to be prayed over (James 5:14)? Of course, that scripture assumes you have elders that believe in healing and know how to pray effectively.

If you don't believe God's will is for healing today, why do you pray for it? So it will manifest in heaven? That's nothing but wasted breath. That's the least needed prayer you can ever pray. Health is automatic in heaven because there's no sin and no fallen nature in heaven. Your health will be perfect for eternity, no prayer required. Why then have we been instructed in the Bible to pray for healing here and now? Isn't it obvious? God wants you well here and now.

> Therefore, let us approach the throne of grace with boldness, so that we may receive mercy and find grace to help us in time of need. - Hebrews 4:16 CSB

Being ill is definitely a *time of need*. Over and over the Bible tells us we will see the goodness of God in the land of the living — yes, right here on earth (Psalm 27:13). His goodness manifested in their lives, even in Old Testament times. Now, in the New Covenant, it should be a given, an assumption, an **expectation** of all believers. Why? Because the Holy Spirit lives in us.

> But if the Spirit of him that raised up Jesus from the dead dwell in you, he that raised up Christ from the dead shall also quicken your **mortal** bodies by his Spirit that dwelleth in you. - Romans 8:11 KJV

If you want to argue that the quickening of our *mortal bodies* refers to the fact that we were born, let me bring to your attention that Paul was writing to people that were already alive, and this verse says SHALL (future tense). The website *www.quora.com* says: "The word *quicken*... means *revive or make alive*. If something is living, it is *quick*; to *quicken* something is to bring it to life or **restore it to a former flourishing condition**." Seriously, folks — how much clearer can God be?

Jesus Himself told us that He came to give us the abundant life. If there is illness in your body, you are not living the abundant life. He also told you to pray for the attributes of heaven to be manifested here on earth. One of those attributes is perfect, divine health. There's no sickness in heaven. We know this. So your health is God's will, and you are instructed to pray that His will is done here on earth. You may have been praying this prayer your whole life, never really meaning it.

> "And he said unto them, Verily I say unto you, There is no man that hath left house, or parents, or brethren, or wife, or children, for the kingdom of God's sake, who shall not receive manifold more in this present time, and in the world to come, life everlasting." - Luke 18:29 KJV

This passage talks about the blessings you obtain here on this earth for sacrifices you make for the sake of God's kingdom. It describes these blessings as *manifold more* (than your sacrifices) in this PRESENT time, AND eternal life. Jesus was speaking regarding Jews still under the law since Jesus had not yet made the ultimate sacrifice. So as a New Covenant believer, you have an even better deal now. The point, though, is that BLESSINGS ARE FOR NOW. In heaven, everything is already blessed.

If what was done on the cross wasn't supposed to affect your life and body here on earth, then all God had to say in the Bible is, "Whatever happens to you in this life, deal with it. When you get to heaven everything will be perfect." But that's not what He said, is it? He inspired thousands of pages about how much He loves you and how He will rescue you out of every adversity. If you don't think disease is adversity, you've never been sick.

Why Would You Receive Healing on Arrival in Heaven When You've Left Your Body Here?

God talks a lot in the Bible of our inheritance in Him. If you can accept that healing is part of your inheritance in Christ, then you will appreciate this nugget. When do you receive an inheritance? Not when YOU die! You receive it when the testator dies, which Jesus did for you two thousand years ago. You receive your inheritance while you're still alive. This is so simple, you need a theologian to help you misunderstand it.

Why did God tell us about Jesus' healings and miracles — in fact why would Jesus even bother to do those miracles if they're not for here and now? To prove his deity? I don't think so. The Father, at Jesus' baptism, sending the visible Holy Spirit and speaking aloud from heaven was all the sign needed to prove Jesus' deity (not to mention over 500 fulfilled prophecies). All He had to do was say, "See all this suffering around you? It won't be like this in Heaven. Believe on Me and join Me in Paradise." But no, He healed them all.

We talked about the wording of Isaiah 53:5 already, but I didn't mention the use of the Greek perfect tense. Perfect tense indicates an ongoing outcome from a previous event. His scourging, humiliation, crown of thorns, crucifixion and resurrection all have ongoing effects, according to the Greek text. They happened centuries ago but continue to provide for us. No translation says *will someday be healed*. It's already been done. The *Amplified Classic Edition* translates it this way:

> But He was wounded for our transgressions, He was bruised for our guilt and iniquities; the chastisement (needful to obtain) of peace and well-being for us was upon Him, and with His stripes (that wounded Him) we are healed and made whole. - Isaiah 53:5 AMPC

What a beautiful verse. What a beautiful Savior.

But That Was Jesus

Maybe you're thinking that you haven't been healed because Jesus isn't here on earth to heal you Himself. Is it different now that He's in heaven? You bet!

> But I tell you the truth, it is to your advantage that I go away… - John 16:7 NASB

> …Blessed *and* happy *and* to be envied are those who have never seen Me and yet have believed *and* adhered to *and* trusted *and* relied on Me. - John 20:29 AMPC

You are enviable! You're mightily blessed when you believe in Jesus today by faith, without the proof of your eyes. If you're sick, what would bless you? Obviously, healing is what would bless you most. Just in case you're subconsciously wondering if He really can do it without His physical presence, remember the story in Matthew 8 of the Roman centurion, a Gentile no less, beseeching Jesus to heal his paralyzed servant. When Jesus offered to accompany the centurion home, the officer replied (paraphrased), "I'm not worthy for you to come to my home. But I understand authority, and if you speak healing regarding my servant, he will be healed." That's faith! The centurion impressed Jesus, and He uses this example to this day in the Bible to demonstrate to us how authority works and to show us that He needn't be physically present for healing.

> "I can guarantee this truth: Those who believe in me will do the things that I am doing. They will do even greater things because I am going to the Father. - John 14:12 GW

So you're supposed to be receiving as if He's speaking healing over you Himself, which He is even though He's not physically present. And you're supposed to carry on His work because He said anyone who believes will also do the things He did. Acts 5 tells you that after Jesus went to the Father, the disciples *healed them all*. That's noteworthy — **the success rate didn't drop after Jesus left.** How was this possible? The disciples were among those who received the Holy Spirit on the day of Pentecost, just as Jesus received the Holy Spirit the day He was baptized and began His ministry. That very same Holy Spirit resides in you. Think about that! Or, in scriptural language: *Selah.*

Not only has Father God demonstrated to you through Jesus that it's His will that you be healed and whole, and that Jesus doesn't have to be present for healing to take place, and that as believers we are supposed to be healing others in the power of the Holy Spirit, He has also assured you that none of this will change. He guarantees it.

> Because God wanted to make the unchanging nature of his purpose very clear to the heirs of what was promised, he confirmed it with an oath. - Hebrews 6:17 NIV

> Jesus Christ is the same yesterday and today and forever. - Hebrews 13:8 NIV

> Who has performed and done this, calling forth [and guiding the destinies of] the generations [of the nations] from the beginning? 'I, the Lord— the first, and with the last [existing before history began, the ever-present, unchanging God]—I am He.' - Isaiah 41:4 AMP

> And the four living creatures, each one of them having six wings, are full of eyes all over and within [underneath their wings]; and day and night they never stop saying, "Holy, holy, holy [is the] Lord God, the Almighty [the Omnipotent, the Ruler of all], who was and who is and who is to come [the unchanging, eternal God]."
> - Revelation 4:8 AMP

He never changes.

> Therefore, let us approach the throne of grace with boldness, so that we may receive mercy and find grace to help us in time of need. - Hebrews 4:16 CSB

Is this your time of need?

Miracles Died with the Apostles
Aka Cessationism

Let's talk about cessationism. To those who contend that healing has passed away (also tongues, prophecy and other gifts of the Spirit), my short answer is this: if healing has passed away then God is dead, too, because His name is Jehovah Rapha — our God who heals.

The term *cessationism* is based on the word *cease*. There are so many shades of cessationism that it's difficult to address the entirety of this subject in one chapter. I tried, and the chapter was so long and bogged down that my editor and I are doing you a favor by stripping it down to the core issues. I'd say that this belief centers on two things: 1) the definition of what constitutes apostleship because cessationists believe only apostles could heal, and 2) the belief that because we now have the New Testament in print, we no longer need the Gifts of the Spirit.

I'll give you the basic parameters of cessationism in point form, and we'll see how they hold up in a quick comparison to the scriptures. Then we'll address the overall subject from a personal, practical, anecdotal perspective instead of a theological one. Yay! That's much more fun.

If you're a die-hard cessationist, know that I am not making light of your beliefs. I take this subject quite seriously. I hope you'll give the information I'm presenting here just as much consideration — your life may depend on it.

The Gifts, Signs and Wonders

Gifts of the Spirit comprise these nine: 1) word of wisdom, 2) word of knowledge, 3) gift of faith (courageous faith usually for application to a specific crisis), 4) gifts of healings, 5) working of miracles, 6) prophecy, 7) discerning of spirits, 8) diversity of tongues and 9) interpretation of tongues (1 Corinthians 12:8-10). You may hear these referred to as the apostolic gifts, sign gifts, manifestation gifts or charismatic gifts, just in case the subject isn't confusing enough on its own. Signs and wonders are the result of these gifts in action. Healing in particular authenticates the gospel because it is often immediately known — the pain vanishes, the limb grows out, the person walks or can hear again, etc. And it makes God's love for you so real. The other gifts can also be used in evangelism — a word of knowledge is often all that is needed to prove God is real and active today.

Cessationists generally hold one of these three positions regarding the gifts:

- They ceased at the end of the *Apostolic Age* (when all the original apostles died).
- They faded away over the next three hundred or so years.
- They ended when the scriptures were canonized (when the Bible was compiled and declared complete and inerrant).
- Further, and sometimes in opposition to the above, cessationists believe either that
- all apostolic gifts are now defunct,
- these things still occur but only in areas of the world where the Gospel has not yet been preached, or
- God still does miracles occasionally but not through people, only sovereignly.

I'm going to answer each of these positions in this book or chapter — indeed, some have already been answered. But first, the reason a cessationist would find it impossible to convert me to their belief is a very simple one. When I look back over the list of spiritual gifts, I don't think there's a single one that I haven't either received or ministered. There was usually another person involved, and I've never lived in an area where the gospel has never been preached.

I literally have a book's worth of miracles and healings recorded. My steps have been directed and my broken heart healed by prayers over me that brought words of wisdom or knowledge or prophecy. Words spoken about this book by a stranger who had no idea I was an author, supplied the encouragement to bring what you're reading right now to fruition. My life has been saved numerous times either by healings or the suspension of natural laws. (I wonder how many times I've been rescued that I'm not even aware of?) I have laid hands on people, and they have been healed. I have cast out demons. I have watched the bed-ridden gain strength and walk within ten minutes of prayer after years of atrophy. I know three people who were raised from the dead, and one was my best friend.

There is absolutely nothing special about me. My friends and family would readily confirm that. So if you do not experience God's power in these ways, then I suspect the only difference between you and me is that I expect to, because there is absolutely something special about our God. There is no way to prove to you that the gifts of the spirit are in operation today if you are dead set against the idea, other than to lay hands on you and heal you. The closest I can come in this book is to share the fact that I have experienced the gifts many times in many ways and hope that for your sake you give God a chance to prove to you that his miraculous power is available to you 24/7.

Regarding the idea of some cessationists that the gifts still occur in remote areas where the gospel has never yet been preached, to authenticate the gospel with signs and wonders, I agree! Just not to the exclusionary clause. God wants EVERYONE saved and loves us all the same. The gifts are in evidence all over the world, every day, in and for people of all kinds. There are people living in the Bible Belt who have never heard the gospel. They're not off God's radar simply because they live in a "Christian nation." God is no respecter of persons. If He'll demonstrate His power for an indigenous person in uncharted territory who has never heard the name of Jesus, He'll do it for you.

These cessationist beliefs about the gifts presuppose that the ONLY reason for the gifts is to authenticate the gospel, which is not true. 1 Corinthians 12 states that they are for the good of ALL. It goes on to speak about the five-fold ministry within the church, so it's obvious the gifts were intended for use within Christ's church. Personally, and based on experience, I believe that everything God gives us is for the benefit of everyone present and everyone that will hear of a specific demonstration of His power because God so loved the WORLD.

As to the notion that God occasionally does miracles without employing humans, this is true, albeit only when we invite Him into the situation through prayer (see the Chapter on sovereignty). But many more workings are done by human hands. It's why we are called the "hands and feet of Jesus." We are told to heal the sick, cast out demons, cleanse the lepers and raise the dead. I suppose a cessationist would say that we weren't told to do that — that Jesus was speaking only to the Apostles at the time. Yes, He was, and He told those Apostles to go and make disciples, teaching them to do everything they'd been instructed to do. That would have included making more disciples. So generation after generation of disciples lead up to today, and we're still supposed to be doing exactly what Jesus instructed the original twelve.

Regarding the middle-of-the-road belief that the Gifts dissipated over three hundred or so years after the apostles died, I can get behind that — the dissipating part, but not to the point of extinction. The dissipating part is still in evidence today. Not because the power was retracted, but because the people were being taught cessationism. And think about this...how can you say that only the Twelve Apostles healed, which is a basic tenet of cessationism, AND that the ability to heal declined over the three hundred years after the apostles died?

The Apostles

Jesus was used by God to heal people. The original apostles and Paul were used by God to heal people. On these statements I don't think there has ever been any dispute. Today, most cessationists believe that to be an apostle one must

- have seen Jesus in resurrected form AND
- have been commissioned by Him personally.

They believe that only the original twelve disciples, minus Judas, plus possibly Matthias who replaced Judas, and Paul, could perform miracles and healings after Jesus' ascension. That would make the Office of Apostle no longer in effect (referring to 1 Corinthians 12:28 and to the five-fold ministry of Ephesians 4:11-16).

The original disciples, when they needed to replace Judas, looked for one who had been with them all along (Acts 1:21, 22) so as to be a witness of Jesus' resurrection. However, sticking to that definition would have excluded Paul. So they had to devise a definition that would include Paul because, well, how could you not include Paul, right? But by including Paul, they've included many others even though these are not acknowledged. Even Paul and the original disciples don't agree with the cessationists' definition of an apostle. There were many others they referred to as apostles.

Conflicting with the cessationist definition, Cruden's Complete Concordance to the Old & New Testaments (revised 1979) defines the word apostle as

1. Literally, one sent forth.
2. Used as referring chiefly to one of the twelve disciples of Christ: (Matthew 10:12); or to **various other followers of Christ who did evangelistic work.**

Over seventy men are called apostles in the Bible, but not by cessationists:

- *The Seventy* were **sent out by Jesus** and given **power over every evil work** (Luke 10: 1, 8-9) — that is the very definition of an **apostle**. Most Protestant Bibles refer to them as disciples, but Eastern Bibles call them the *Seventy Apostles*. Note that in 1 Corinthians 15:5, 6, Paul reports the resurrected Jesus met with the twelve and then with ALL the **Apostles** at a later date. This is referring to the seventy, and perhaps others.
- Ananias — The Bible calls Ananias an **apostle**, so to justify that, some cessationists claim he replaced the deceased James — but there's no scripture to back up that claim AND James died long after Paul was saved. So if Ananias replaced James and became an *official* apostle, he did so long after he ministered healing, prophecy and baptism to Paul (Acts 22:12-19).
- Barnabas — Barnabas was sent by the Holy Spirit to minister in Asia Minor (Acts 13) placing him square in the role of apostle. The Bible refers to him as an **apostle** (Acts 11:22-26), but he didn't make the cessationists' list.
- Apollos — Paul refers to him as an **apostle** (1 Corinthians 3: 4).
- Andronicus and Junia — Paul said, "Salute Andronicus and Junia, my kinsmen, and my fellow prisoners, who are **of note among the apostles**, who also were in Christ before me" (Romans 16:7 KJV).
- Titus and two brethren — They were called *messengers of the churches* (2 Corinthians 8)—the Greek word is *apostello*, which means **apostles**.
- Epaphroditus—The **apostle** sent from the church at Philippi to care for Paul when he was under house arrest in Jerusalem (Philippians 2:25-30)

Remember that cessationists believe that only apostles could heal and perform miracles.

> And God has appointed these in the church: first apostles, second prophets, third teachers, after that miracles, then gifts of healings, helps, administrations, varieties of tongues.
> - 1 Corinthians 12:28 NKJV

The scripture above does not limit miracle-working to apostles. Below are some that are not known as apostles but are specifically mentioned in the Bible as performing demonstrations of the power of God, with total disregard for the cessationist belief system. No doubt there were more.

- Stephen — the first Christian martyr, whose death marked the beginning of the great persecution of the church in Jerusalem — "Stephen, full of grace and power, was **performing great wonders and signs** among the people" (Acts 6:8).
- Philip the deacon (Acts 8:5-7) — This Philip was not referred to as an apostle, yet he traveled to preach; he **healed and delivered** the people of Samaria establishing the Gospel there —the very definition of apostleship.
- Timothy and Silas/Silvanus — not called apostles but **served as apostles** would have; they traveled with Paul preaching, **healing**, making disciples, risking life and limb for the gospel (1 Corinthians) and co-authoring a couple of epistles.

There is no scriptural basis for limiting the list of apostles to Paul and the eleven or twelve. And it's quite obvious that **not** only the twelve and Paul could minister healing. But how does proving that cessationism is not scriptural as regards Biblical times, have any impact on our lives today?

Here's how: if cessationism is in error, then the Gifts haven't passed away — they're still in operation today, and YOU can use them. Fact: cessationists are mistaken according to scripture and according to the real-life experiences of many Christians even today, including myself.

In reality, we know that it's not apostles that perform miracles, it's the Holy Spirit — the same Holy Spirit that has been at every dead-raising from the beginning of time, including Jesus'. And that Spirit is the same one that makes His dwelling place inside each and every believer, including you. How could anyone think He's chosen to stop doing what He tells you is His nature when He also tells you He does not change?

> Heal the sick who are there and tell them, 'The kingdom of God is near you.' - Luke 10:9 BSB

Healing manifests when sickness is confronted by the Kingdom of God. How does the Kingdom come near to you? The same way it did when Jesus sent out the seventy. The Kingdom is inside every believer. Jesus delegated authority to the twelve and the seventy, and perhaps others as He is recorded as having met with five hundred after His resurrection. But today, we have inherited authority because we have the Holy Spirit— you carry Him with you. You carry Him into every situation, circumstance, and hospital room you enter. The Kingdom is there for you to walk in, access, and put to use with authority over every work of the devil the same way Jesus did, for yourself and for others.

> The Spirit's presence is shown in some way in each person for the good of all. - 1 Corinthians 12:7 GNT

Each person — no mention of apostles there.

THE Obvious Answer to Cessationism vs Continuationism

As I was finishing up the first run at writing this chapter — many more pages than you now see — a link caught my eye on a recent search screen. It was for a John Piper teaching on cessationism vs. continuationism, touted as being a well-rounded, unbiased look at both sides of the subject. Based on that description, I decided to take the time to watch it. Piper was described in the write-up as a Reformed Baptist and a continuationist who also defends the uniqueness of both the apostles and the socio-political and religious climate of that historical period. Here is his own description, from the video, of the two camps:

Cessationism: We shouldn't seek signs and miracles because they were only granted in Jesus' day to prove what we now have enshrined in the New Testament — a unique apostolic authority.
Continuationism: Signs and wonders ARE for today. We don't experience more of them because we don't expect them, but they should be sought for the sake of blessing the church and empowering evangelism.

This sounded very promising — practical, down-to-earth, rubber-meets-the-road descriptions — so far, so good. Then he said that he reads books and combs scripture; he prays and agonizes and still finds himself teetering back and forth between the two. My immediate reaction was to stop the video and get back to writing. I wasn't going to waste my time.

What had I just heard that made me turn off the video? Did you catch it? Piper had indicated that he was open to whichever camp held the truth, but he just couldn't figure out which one that was. Think about the descriptions he gave of the two points of view — don't seek signs and miracles because they don't happen today versus expect them and they will happen. He's had his answer for years, right there in front of him: seek and expect them!

If you step out on a limb and earnestly expect God to show up and take part in your life and ministry by backing you up with demonstrations of His power and He says, "No," it won't make Him any less God. It will only define what we can ask of Him today. If signs and wonders are not for today, then they won't happen no matter how much you expect them. If you start from a position of insisting signs and wonders are not for today, I guarantee you they won't happen, because faith, your earnest expectation, is required for miracles to happen.

From personal experience and that of friends and acquaintances, I can assure you that today God is everything the Bible shows Him to have been. He never changes. When you give God permission to handle what life throws at you anyway He sees fit, you're going to see miracles. When you tell Him, "I don't see a way out of this situation, but I know You ARE the Way," you will see miracles. When you say, "Lord I don't know how You're going to fix this, but I know you've already done it," you will see miracles.

You know, the Bible says we shall have ANYTHING within His will that we ask of Him in faith, and healing is very near the top of His list of favorite things. So EXPECT your healing to manifest because it has already been done. I cannot answer for every past time you wanted a miracle or healing and it didn't happen, at least not without some information. Usually it's because we give up, allowing our five senses to influence us instead of God's Word. I do it, too.

Don't let your past determine your future. I've experienced too many healings and miracles in my own life — received, observed, and ministered — to ever believe otherwise. There's just no denying that God is a continuationist. He continues to be the same yesterday, today, and forever.

The Great Commission on Your Life Continuationism in Action

To me, it is telling that the church overall labels Matthew's description of that day as The Great Commission, rather than Mark's. This was the day of Jesus' ascension into heaven, and these are His final instructions to the disciples — pretty important stuff. Mark 16 tells us more about what Jesus said that day, and in doing so, gives us more understanding about the power and authority Jesus has entrusted us with. It also places more responsibility on us to use that power and authority. Jesus, that day, told us all to go and preach the gospel and make disciples of all nations.

A disciple is a student who learns from a specific teacher and models that teacher's beliefs and actions. So all apostles have been and are disciples, but not all disciples are apostles. Except that they are supposed to

> You Are Called to Be an Apostle

be. Because that day Jesus called you, , He sent you — as *Cruden's* described, *"literally, one sent forth."*

Another definition of apostle is "a vigorous and pioneering advocate or supporter of a particular policy, idea, or cause." (Google Dictionary, s.v., "apostle," accessed (June 20, 2020), *http://www.googledictionary.com/apostle*) We all should certainly be that as regards our faith.

Disciples do exactly what the person teaching them does, and so a disciple must make disciples of his own, and again, teach them to duplicate the process of making disciples. That means that, by the basic definitions, we are all called to be apostles because we are all called to go and make disciples, according to the Great Commission:

> Jesus came near and said to them, "All authority has been given to me in heaven and on earth. Go, therefore, and make disciples of all nations, baptizing them in the name of the Father and of the Son and of the Holy Spirit, teaching them to **observe everything I have commanded you**. And remember, I am with you always, to the end of the age." - Matthew 28: 16-20 CSB

> Later he appeared to the Eleven themselves as they were reclining at the table. He rebuked their unbelief and hardness of heart, because they did not believe those who saw him after he had risen. Then he said to them, "Go into all the world and preach the gospel to all creation. Whoever believes and is baptized will be saved, but whoever does not believe will be condemned. And these signs will accompany those who believe: In my name they will drive out demons; they will speak in new tongues; they will pick up snakes; if they should drink anything deadly, it will not harm them; they will lay hands on the sick, and they will get well."
> - Mark 16:14-18 CSB

How could Jesus make it more clear? But let's break it down anyway because I want to be certain nobody misses this. There were the original disciples — let's call them generation one of Christ's followers. Then those who were saved during the ministry of Jesus and His disciples — generation two. Scripture has proven that generation two did the same things generation one did, preaching the Kingdom and demonstrating the power of God, getting people saved, and discipling them. This group would have included the seventy. The first two generations were to get baptized in the Holy Spirit, then go forth to all the earth and make generation three, right? We know this because we know there were over a hundred people in the Upper Room at Pentecost.

Who are *those who believe* in Matthew 28 and Mark 16? Is that just the eleven disciples? Obviously not. It is those to whom the gospel is preached BY generations one and two and who accept it. *Those who believe* are generation three. These would be the post-ascension generation of believers. They may never have seen Jesus alive.

Note that Jesus is telling the eleven to preach to the entire human race. Does any Christian think this commission to spread the Gospel applies to only the Apostles or only to the generation three — that only people alive when Christ ascended were to be offered salvation? No Christian believes that. We all know it applies to us today… generation after generation. Then the rest of the passage applies to us today as well, so *those who believe* has to include today's believers.

And the apostles were to teach generation three to do the exact same things — receive the gospel, go and preach it, demonstrate God's power to authenticate it, serve people with compassion, and make disciples. Repeat. Repeat. Repeat.

Are You A Believing Believer?

Do you see that if Jesus had any intention of withdrawing the power (the Holy Spirit) from men, then He could not have given the instructions in The Great Commission — even in Matthew's account. He even said He would be with us until the end of the age, and we're still in that same age. Another perspective is this. If signs and wonders cannot follow believers today, then Jesus is a liar because He said for us to make disciples and teach them to do everything He and the apostles did.

Therefore, today's believers will be accompanied by those attesting signs. In other words, any **believer** that you ask to pray for you, will lay hands on you and you will get well. At least, that is how it is supposed to work. We're all supposed to be in faith. We're supposed to EXPECT healing and every good thing. Further, if you're a Christian and you've never laid hands on another person EXPECTING healing to occur, you need to rectify that according to scripture. Note that this command applies to **believers**. Do you qualify? Unfortunately, today we have to qualify Christians because so many of us believe Jesus is the Son of God Who redeemed us, but **we don't believe what our Lord and Savior says**! He says attesting signs will follow you if you believe.

Jesus specifically commissioned the twelve disciples and the seventy, because the Holy Spirit had not yet come. Once Jesus ascended and Pentecost took place, that power was suddenly available to all who believed, so Jesus in bodily form giving you a specific commission and granting of power and authority to individuals is not needed. This is why He went to the Father — so that the Holy Spirit could come and dwell in us, embolden and empower us.

This does not mean that you have to go on a mission trip or move to Togo to fulfill The Great Commission. It does not mean you're called to the Office of Apostle within the church (reference the Five-Fold Ministry of Ephesians 4:11). But, you do have your own sphere of influence, and every believer is called to ministry, to make disciples, to act as apostle in the basic definition — one who is sent. Jesus said we are to renew our minds, love God, love one another, speak in tongues, lay hands on the sick, cast out demons, and raise the dead. He will protect us from harm — from devils, from snakebite and poison, from every sickness, and He set angels to encamp about us and guard us so that we don't even stub our toes. So, go heal the sick, make disciples, and in the doing, receive your own healing.

CHAPTER 11
Unworthiness

I'm Not Worthy

You're right. You're not, not in and of yourself. Neither am I. Neither is your spouse, kids (regardless of age), parents, church leaders — none but Jesus is worthy.

If you are saved, though, it doesn't matter how bad your past or even present is, Jesus makes you flawless in God's eyes, worthy of all His blessings — worthy of healing. Of course, it's not due to your own works but because of Jesus'. This is because you are IN Christ. Everything that is Jesus' is yours! So do not fall for those lying whispers, telling you that healing is not for you because you're not deserving of it. None of us is deserving of it, but we're made worthy by Jesus. That's why it's a gift, a blessing, part of God's grace available to us all. You cannot earn it, so your unworthiness is moot. You have a new identity in Christ, and that identity makes you worthy.

Scripture shows there were no conditions placed on being healed. Jesus never even told the sick to confess first. He already knew their sins, and He healed them anyway. God heals the unworthy because He loves us all the same. These days, unbelievers get healed all the time. Street healers walk around like mini Jesuses (as we're all supposed to) and minister healing to unbelievers almost exclusively. When these unbelievers get healed, they often get saved. God is so good.

God heals you partly because His goodness draws you to Him and leads you to repentance — to change your mind toward Him or about Him. And there's even more good news.

> But by His doing you are in Christ Jesus, who became to us wisdom from God, and righteousness and sanctification, and redemption, - 1 Corinthians 1:30 NASB

> Because of our faith, Christ has brought us into this place of undeserved privilege where we now stand, and we confidently and joyfully look forward to sharing God's glory. - Romans 5:2 NLT

It has nothing to do with anything you have done. This means that there's nothing you CAN do — **you are relieved of responsibility as to the provision of healing.** You are IN Jesus as a Christian. You are one with Him. Even though you don't deserve anything good, Jesus does, and because He placed you in Him, whatever He receives so do you. The instant you are born again, every blessing and promise of God that's in the Bible becomes yours because you are in Christ.

Unworthiness Is Moot — Healing was Bequeathed to You Long Before You Were Born

Let's use the analogy of a Last Will and Testament again. Say your earthly dad has a will, and you are named as his heir. It's a lot of money. When do you get it? When the testator, in this case your dad, passes away. Were you the perfect child and therefore, deserve it? No, you probably rebelled, didn't go into the family business, and dated the antithesis of the person your parents pictured as your future spouse. But you're his child and he loves you, so he made you his heir. Did you earn any of the money in this inheritance? Not a cent. Your dad worked for every penny. But is it still yours? Yes, it's yours, legally yours — yours to do with as you like. You can ignore it and let it sit in a bank account and never access it, or you can withdraw any of it at any time. It's yours. Do you question if it's yours or not? Every time you go to the bank, do you get the teller to verify that your name is still on the account? No! You know it's yours because you're a child of the testator.

Your spiritual inheritance works much the same way as an earthly one, except that you can never withdraw it all. It's endless, infinite. Did Jesus die? Yes, He died to give you this inheritance that He obtained for you. Did you do anything to earn it? Or even to deserve it? No, Jesus did it all. Nonetheless, it is yours. You inherited it — the whole enchilada. You never need question it, because it's yours forever. Nobody can take it away from you because it's legally yours. What did you inherit? Peace, provision, protection, joy, the blessing of Abraham, the right to call on every attribute in every name of God, every promise and every blessing in the scriptures. Healing is YOURS! It's been yours since Jesus died because He willed it to you.

So, your unworthiness is immaterial because:
- You can't earn it — it's a gift, no strings attached;
- Jesus heals both saints and sinners—it's just Who He is;
- Jesus paid for it already so you may as well take it; and
- It's your inheritance — you're a joint heir with Christ.

I Must Have Done Something Wrong

The *you get what you deserve* mentality permeates our culture. Karma. But that's not how Christianity works.

As a child, I remember seeing *The Sound of Music* for the first time, and Julie Andrews singing "Something Good"

Karma and New Covenant Christianity Are Incompatible

with Christopher Plummer — a song that stated they must have done something really good in their younger days to warrant their newly discovered, reciprocated love. If you believe you get good things because you do good, then it naturally follows that you get bad things when you do bad. It's human nature to nod along knowingly as the character Maria sings about the impossibility of good things happening without doing good.

As a Christ-follower, though, your mindset is supposed to be different than that of our culture, our world. Instead, it should line up with God's way of thinking which is 1) that His grace is a free gift that you cannot earn, 2) that He will never again be angry with us or punish us (Isaiah 54:9), and 3) that Jesus has already paid for our sins. Could you ever have imagined that *The Sound of Music* promotes the lies of the devil? And she's a nun, no less!

God provides for you according to HIS riches in glory in Christ Jesus (Philippians 4:19), not according to what you deserve. We all deserve death (Romans 6:23) because we all sin, and the wages of sin is death. But Christ came, and all that we deserve is now under the Blood of Jesus, praise God.

> For if while we were enemies we were reconciled to God through the death of His Son, it is much more [certain], now that we are reconciled, that we shall be saved (daily delivered from sin's dominion) through His [resurrection] life. - Romans 5:10 AMPC

Everything that makes you deserving of sickness and death has been thrown into the Sea of Forgetfulness (Micah 7:19) and is as far from you as the east is from the west (Psalm 103:12). It no longer has power over you — not even your future sins. Every sin you will ever commit was forgiven two thousand years ago. The Father had full knowledge of every jealous thought, every stolen dollar, every lustful glance, every abortion. He knew it all. He judged it all. He punished it all in advance on the timeless body of Jesus.

> **Say Aloud:**
> **I Am the Righteousness**
> **of God in Christ**
> **(Repeat Many Times Daily)**

For that reason, He cannot punish YOU for it. Our legal system calls it double jeopardy. God cannot punish you for something He already punished Jesus for. If He did, He would be acting unjustly, and His entire reign would crumble because as Psalm 89:14 tells us, the foundation of His Throne is righteousness and justice. And this was all His idea, His plan! Ingenious.

So root out the thought that you are sick due to your OWN sinfulness. You are sick because there is sin in this world and you are just finding out that you are no longer under the curse of that sin. But you are not being punished — Jesus already took your punishment Himself, in his own body, and bled to wash away your sin. You don't deserve illness because you're now the righteousness of God in Christ Jesus regardless of your sins. It is finished. Go and sin no more in grateful response to His love and grace.

My Sin Blocks the Blessings

There's a mindset permeating the Church that our sins will stop God's blessings in our life. "Sure, maybe God wants most people healed, but there are consequences for our actions, you know. He may have forgiven me, but there's no way He can heal me because I've been doing drugs or cheating on my spouse or watching porn or been unable to forgive my sister or falsifying my taxes or had an abortion or (insert sin of your choice), and that's just too bad to be overlooked. It's consequence to bear."

If that were true, how is it that Jesus healed and performed miracles for the prostitutes, the tax collectors, the adulterers and others labeled sinners and outcasts? They were no different from any of us.

Above my husband's bed in the ICU, I could see the two of them — Kevin and Jesus — sitting in Adirondack chairs, talking. I couldn't see the vista they were admiring, but I know it was serene, like sitting on the beach at twilight. They were talking about our son and me. I couldn't make out the words, but I knew the gist of it. Kevin was deciding what to do — go on to heaven or come back into his body. And Jesus was telling him to base that decision on his own desire, because He would take care of our son and me. He had us covered.

"No! Don't tell Kevin that! He won't come back if he thinks I don't need him, and I DO need him!" The next time I saw into the spirit realm, I got even more vehement. "Shut up! Just shut up." Later it got even worse. I have an arsenal of expletives from my former life, and I used them. Yes, I told the Creator of the universe to shut the - - - - up (insert four letters of your choice — whatever they are, I probably used them). We talk about Peter denying Christ WITH CURSING as if that made the action so much worse, when in reality the denial was the deep issue. Let's just say that I left no doubt as to where I stood on the issue of my husband's physical survival. Going BOLDLY before the throne is something I've definitely put into practice!

Friday night, after Kevin passed, I was eventually alone in our hotel room — physically alone for the first time without a husband. My son and his girlfriend had gone for take-out, assuring me they wouldn't be more than thirty minutes. I began to shake with cold and shock, and my feet felt like blocks of ice. They were so cold they burned. I had socks, but I could only get one on. More than a year earlier I had twisted my hip joint, and I couldn't make that inward swinging motion with my leg necessary to put on a sock. Even sitting on the bed, I couldn't bend toward that right foot enough to get a sock on it. Cocooned under the covers, with extra blankets piled on top, my right foot still ached with the cold. So I threw off the covers and snarled at Jesus, "You want to be my husband? Fine. Then GET down here and put this sock on for me because that's what Kevin would do." I was riled up. I never for a moment thought that God TOOK my husband, but I was mad that He didn't tell Kevin to come back for my sake.

So there I was, angry at God, cursing Him, absolutely in a state of sin and not even caring that I was — not a repentant bone to be found anywhere in me. What was the Lord's response? He healed my hip. Right there, sitting alone on the side of a hotel bed, nobody else around to pray over me. I hadn't even asked. He healed me so that I got my sock on without pain that night and every time I've wanted socks on since. It's not that often, as I'm a southern girl, and barefoot is a state of being in the South. But up north here, I have to admit, socks can be needful. And He met my need.

I was full of anger (which He sees as murder), but His heart was still to heal me. That's how much, how deep, and how unconditional His love is for us. Sin cannot stop his love. Sin cannot stop His healing.

> He has not dealt with us according to our sins, nor punished us according to our iniquities, For as the heavens are high above the earth, so great is His mercy toward those who fear Him; as far as the east is from the west, so far has He removed our transgressions from us.
> - Psalm 103:10-12 NKJV

> "Their sins and lawless acts I will remember no more."
> - Hebrews 10:17 NIV

Let me clarify one thing, though. Your continuing in ongoing sin will definitely harm your relationship with God. Not because He will draw away from you, though. It's the opposite — because of your own feelings of guilt and shame and the diminished time you will spend fellowshipping with Him, hiding from Him as Adam and Eve did. But sin itself cannot separate you from His love. Sin has been dealt with.

In the Old Covenant, sin did separate you from God, which is why the priests were always standing, making sacrifices — the work was never done. As He died, Jesus declared, "Finished!" (debt paid in full, work completed, and in military parlance, to declare a battle won). God tore the temple veil, top to bottom, destroying the barrier between Himself and mankind, allowing us free access to the Holy of Holies. And when Jesus ascended to the Father, as our High Priest, He SAT DOWN, an action declaring the sacrifices completed. Finished means finished.

> Now every *cohen* (priest) stands every day doing his service, offering over and over the same sacrifices, which can never take away sins. But this one, after he had offered for all time a single sacrifice for sins, sat down at the right hand of God, from then on to wait until his enemies be made a footstool for his feet. For by a single offering he has brought to the goal for all time those who are being set apart for God and made holy. - Hebrews 10:11-14 CJB

Brought to the goal... TOUCHDOWN!

> Now where remission of these *is, there is* no more offering for sin. *then He adds,* "Their sins and their lawless deeds I will remember no more." - Hebrews 10:17, 18 NKJV

AND THE CROWD GOES WILD...We're told now to:

...come boldly before the throne of Grace, that we may obtain mercy and find grace to help in time of need.
- Hebrews 4:16 NKJV

So, brothers, we have confidence to use the way into the Holiest Place opened by the blood of Yeshua. (Jesus)
- Hebrews 10:19 CJB

We need God's grace all day, every day. Do we ever deserve it? No. Even when we're not sinning, when everything's going great in our lives, we still fall far short of God's excellence. But when we've just blown it, when we're sick, when we're struggling with something, we really feel the need for grace. Perfect timing, since it is the UNDESERVED, UNMERITED, UNEARNED favor of God.

We must believe God's Word. He chooses His words wisely, because He is bound to uphold them. He doesn't tell us we're free from the condemnation that prevents the flow of His blessing to us if it's not true. By one offering — the sacrifice of Jesus — you have been perfected! God sees you IN Jesus. Your spirit is flawless once you accept Him, because the Holy Spirit enters you, and God, being spirit, relates to you in spirit. Nothing you do in the entirety of your life can cause you to be out of fellowship with God, unless you pull away from him through condemnation you put on yourself. He loves you without a single string attached and wants to commune with you no matter the state you're in. Yes, you can stop God's blessings in your life — not by your sin, but by your unbelief or self-condemnation.

Grace - by Definition - Is ONLY for those Who Don't Deserve It

Remember that God is the same yesterday, today and forever and is no respecter of persons. The tax collectors and prostitutes and everyday citizens in Jesus' day weren't even Christians yet! They only had the blood of bulls and goats. Their sins had been swept under the rug, but not paid for and sent as far as the east is from the west.

You have far better standing with God than did those prior to Jesus' death and resurrection. That means you have far better standing with God than they did when Jesus healed them! Are your sins bad? Yes. Do they deserve to be punished? They're punishable by death. That's the point. Jesus stood in for you. He took your punishment. With that in mind, do you really want to carry on in adultery? Are you having second thought about those funds you're embezzling? Have you asked forgiveness for that abortion? Then it's finished. Take your healing, and live a life of gratitude for what He did for you. And make sure you don't waste His work at the cross — accept all the gifts He gave you!

> If the death of his Son restored our relationship with God while we were still his enemies, we are even more certain that, because of this restored relationship, the life of his Son will save (**sozo**) us. - Romans 5:10 GW

Do you really think what you did wrong is bigger than what Jesus did at the cross? You're just not that important. Next time you fall short, satan's minions will again whisper, "Think about what you've done. How can you call yourself a Christian? God can't heal a sinner like you." You just tell them, "It's covered by the Blood!"

He's Teaching Me a Lesson (Disciplining Me in Love)

Do you hear God's voice? Can you read His instruction in the Bible? If you can do either or both of these, why would He need to do you harm to teach you? If you don't hear Him, then He wants you to draw nearer to Him so that you come to understand Him clearly. The Bible tells us it's His goodness that draws us near, not fear of thinking that He'll make you sick. I don't know about you, but that would repel me. Why would anyone want to worship a God who harmed them? Would you give your child a disease or break his leg to teach him something? Of course not. There are special places with bars for parents like that. And even there, anyone who harms a child has to be separated from the murderers and rapists and thieves for their own bodily protection. Even felons know that anyone who would harm a child is deserving of a special kind of hell. That description does not fit our God. What kind of father would that make Him?

Stop Accusing God of Child Abuse!

Some people think God uses illness when we need *tough love*. With your wayward, willful child, you just have to take the hard line, right? Here are some definitions of the term *tough love*.
- love or affectionate concern expressed in a stern or unsentimental manner (as through discipline) especially to promote responsible behavior *(Merriam-Webster https://www.merriam-webster.com)*

- the practice of being very strict with someone in order to help them overcome a problem with their behavior.
  (https://www.collinsdictionary.com/us/dictionary/english)
- the fact of deliberately not showing too much kindness to a person who has a problem so that the person will start to solve their own problems *(Cambridge English Dictionary* or *https://dictionary.cambridge.org/us)*
- strict discipline or imposing specific obligations or requirements on a person to mandate responsibility *(https://www.yourdictionary.com)*

There is no mention of bodily harm in any definition of *tough love*. Should we make good decisions and behave well? Of course. But when you don't, Jesus has already taken responsibility for your actions. They have been paid for.

Let me give you another slightly different perspective on this. If you, like so many parents today, feel corporal punishment at school or at home is wrong, even equating it with child abuse, how can you think that God would use it on you? How can you glorify God for making you suffer something you believe is dead wrong?

Another point: God wants you leaning *not on your own understanding* but on Him in your everyday life. I fail to see how illness coming from God would turn a person toward Him or improve their relationship. Again, it's His goodness that draws us to Him.

Our Heavenly Father is infinite and has so very many ways to teach, discipline, lead, guide, and correct you. There's no need for bodily harm. What is God's primary way of disciplining, teaching, leading and guiding? His Word, the Holy Bible, is.

Another, somewhat more palatable and related belief, is that healing can come, but the Lord's going to make sure you learn the spiritual lessons He wants you to understand before He'll heal you. You know, I've yet to find a sick person that can tell me what God is trying to teach them when they're ill. What spiritual lesson would you learn from God giving you a disease? Or from delaying a healing? Perhaps that He doesn't love you as much as you hoped? I can't find any spiritual lesson to be taught through sickness. No wait — I retract that statement. Jesus did teach something before He healed, and Paul did the same. They taught that your sins are forgiven so that you can have faith

> God's GOODNESS Draws Us to Him — We Are Not Drawn if We Think He'll Make Us Sick

to receive healing! The one thing He wants you to learn when you're sick — that healing is His will for you!

God does not need to use infirmity to teach you or discipline you. If you are sick and broken, will He use it in some way? Yes. He can turn ALL things to good (Romans 8:28). He will put just the right scriptures and teaching materials in front of you to make use of your down time. He will send just the right visitors to you with just the right word for You if you will receive it. He will give you rest if that's what you need. (But please realize that rest when you're ill is not nearly as productive as rest when you're healthy. Most of that rest is directed toward making you well rather than recharging your batteries.) He will give you doctors, nurses and hospital roommates that need to hear the gospel and see you get out of that bed healthy by His power. There are many ways He can put it to use — ways we can't even fathom. But He does not create the situation.

I heard a woman testify once that she was ill one day, feeling just awful. The next day her middle child complained of the same symptoms, so she kept him home from school. That day, her toddler got a belt wrapped around her neck somehow, then stumbled on the steps, and freakishly ended up dangling by the belt, strangling. The middle child, who normally would have been at school, saw her and lifted her, saving her life. The family thanked God for the boy's illness, the reason he was home that day. The mother asked God why He'd allowed her to be sick the day before, since she knew God didn't want her ill, and she reported that God told her it was so she'd know how terrible the middle child felt and allow him to stay home. Praise God that the toddler survived the day.

Here's the thing — The Lord could just as easily have said to the mom, "The baby's in danger, go downstairs NOW." Or prevented the danger to begin with by saying to the dad, "Don't leave your belt in the stairwell." Or even just steered the toddler supernaturally away from danger in that moment. But God works within the parameters of our faith in that season of our relationship with Him. All we need to do is to trust that, one way or another, He will protect us when He is invited into our everyday lives. Know that His will for us is not to be sick a single day of our lives. How do I know that? Because He paid for our health ahead of time.

You may be reading this book because of a life-threatening condition. But it's God's will that we walk in divine health and never have so much as a headache or a case of the sniffles. No doubt some people stayed home from their office in the Twin Towers due to illness on September 11, 2001, and you can certainly say that the condition was put to good use. But illness is never necessary to God's task of providing everything you need, including discipline and instruction, if you will only hear Him and obey. (I'm preaching to myself here, too!) People didn't have to be sick that

September 11 to avoid death. Many Christians reported running out-of-the-way errands before going to the office, not really knowing why. God is infinite and has infinite ways to teach, guide, correct and direct us. It's all about relationship. He only wants good for you. What decent parent would want otherwise? We read a different translation of this already, but it's a great scripture. After cleansing the world with the Great Flood, God declared:

> "Just as I swore in the time of Noah that I would never again let a flood cover the earth, so now I swear that I will never again be angry and punish you." - Isaiah 54:9 NLT

Know that. Make that your memory verse today. God has sworn that He is not mad at you and will not punish you. Meditate on that and be healed. You are His beloved. He loves you with a perfect love.

> There is no fear in love; instead, perfect love drives out fear, because **fear involves punishment**. So the one who fears is not complete in love. - 1 John 4:18 CSB

Be fearless!

CHAPTER 12
God is Sovereign

We spent an entire chapter on this subject, so you understand the balance between God's dominion and the dominion he gave us on the earth. The following beliefs are the places the human mind goes when it doesn't have a handle on the sovereignty issue.

God Gets the Glory for My Suffering

No doubt you've heard this before — maybe you've even said it. Just how does that work?

When a Christian is ill, no doubt God will put it to use somehow in His infinite wisdom, because the Word tells us that He will turn ALL things to good for those who love Him and are called according to His purpose (Romans 8:28). But do you really think that unbelievers look at Christians and say, "Now I see — God really is good. Look how He has enabled her to endure pain with a smile on her face and a Bible on her lap?" NO! They say, "If God's so good, why hasn't He healed that guy that spouted scriptures all day before he went on sick leave?" And you can be certain there are numerous Christians silently asking the same question.

There are many things I can glorify God for that happened around and after my husband's death, but not the pain he endured, and not the death itself. They were not God's will. God did not take Kevin nor cause his pain — He allowed him to go home even though healing would have brought God the glory that his death did not. Kevin's death wasn't a bad thing for him — he is having a lot more fun than I am right now. I'm ok with that. But what does the world see? They see that my husband died. Period. The end. That does not bring God glory in the world's eyes. If Kevin was here to testify of his miraculous healing, there would be lots more glorifying going on and lots more people turning toward our wonderful God.

> So the crowd marveled as they saw the mute speaking, the crippled restored, and the lame walking, and the blind seeing; and they glorified the God of Israel.
> - Matthew 15:31 NASB

Illness and death do not glorify God — healing does!

> For no matter how many promises God has made, they are "Yes" in Christ. And so through him the "Amen" is spoken by us to the glory of God. - 2 Corinthians 1:20 NIV

God does not get glory for something that comes from satan. Death is called God's enemy in the Bible, and as we've said many times already, sickness and disease are incipient death.

> The thief comes only to steal and kill and destroy. I have come that they may have life (ZOE!), and have it in all its fullness. - John 10:10 BSB

God gets glory when people are healed because everyone sees that God is keeping His promise. The word *glory* in this context just means *a good opinion*. People's opinion of God changes (that's the real meaning of *repent*) when they see Him heal. Do not be fooled. God does not receive any glory whatsoever when you let the devil tromp all over you. Many books have been written that say otherwise, but not a single unbeliever thinks this God stuff may be what he needs when he sees Christians supposedly made to suffer disease and death for their God. And do you know what? Those unbelievers are right, because the god of suffering and disease is the devil.

God's will is *Life*, and He expects you to fight for His will to be executed on earth. You are a co-laborer with Christ. We need to stop letting our idle words and our unbelief, whereby we curse ourselves and agree with the devil, tie God's hands. We are preventing Him, in our own lives, from keeping His promise to be our God that heals us.

Suffering for Jesus

"Well, I'm just sick because I'm suffering with Jesus. The Bible tells us there will be troubles…"

Yes, but He promises to be with us through them. He even promises to deliver us from them ALL.

> Many are the afflictions of the righteous, But the LORD delivers him out of them all. - Psalm 34:19 NKJV

How can that be true when the Bible also says we're supposed to partake of Jesus' suffering? Once again the seeming contradiction in the Bible is no contradiction at all. We ARE to partake of Jesus' suffering, but which suffering? His torturous death was one He volunteered for, to take our punishment. In other words, He did it because He didn't want us to have to. So don't partake of that! The suffering we're to partake in is the suffering of His life, not of His death, and His only suffering in life was persecution for the Gospel.

Jesus was never sick a day in His life! He walked in divine health. Partake of that.

He never lacked anything. The Magi made Him wealthy. His expensive one-piece linen robe was the envy of all the soldiers at His crucifixion. Fish brought him cash to pay taxes with (Matthew 17:27), and women, wives of Romans and others including Mary Magdalene supported Him and the disciples throughout their ministry (Luke 8:1-3). Partake of that.

He had perfect shalom, the peace that passes all understanding and includes every good thing — nothing missing, nothing broken. He bequeathed His shalom to you. Partake of that.

But, aren't we supposed to pick up our cross — suffer with Jesus? Yes, we're to suffer persecution for the sake of His Name and the gospel. Here's more scriptural proof:

> Calling the crowd along with his disciples, he said to them, "If anyone wants to follow after me, let him deny himself, take up his cross, and follow me." - Mark 8:34 CSB

Watch this next verse (emphasis added):

> For whoever wants to save his life will lose it, But whoever loses his life BECAUSE OF ME AND THE GOSPEL will save it. - Mark 8:35 CSB

What does *because of Me and the gospel* mean? Jesus is describing persecution.

> ### Jesus Suffered to Give You Blessings Now —
> ### There Are No Extra Crowns in Heaven for Rejecting Them

He is certainly not talking about sickness. Illness does nothing to promote the gospel — quite the opposite. We're supposed to be examples, lights in the darkness showing forth God's goodness. Being sick does not exemplify God's goodness to the lost world — that's just more of the same to them. Remember that Jesus told the seventy disciples to heal and deliver all people they encountered in order to confirm the gospel.

Let's all learn to be well so that we are better witnesses! The only suffering we are called to as New Covenant Christians is persecution for His Name's sake — for the gospel. He took care of everything else at the cross because everything else results from sin and the curses of Genesis 3 and Deuteronomy 28. Living for Jesus has nothing to do with the curse.

Be sure you always differentiate between illness, and physical suffering due to persecution. The former we are not called to, the latter we possibly could be, to varying degrees. Physical suffering for the gospel is ultimately martyrdom, and offers great rewards. But there's no reward in heaven for ignoring what Jesus suffered to give you. That's the opposite of what God's will is for you, and it brings much of Jesus' suffering to naught. It does not honor Him to refuse what He suffered to give you.

This should simplify it. If Jesus suffered to give it to you, then it's obviously His will for you. Not receiving the healing He took the stripes for is going against His will.

We are supposed to become more and more like Jesus every day, and Jesus was never sick. We are not called to be sick, to be impoverished, to be in lousy marriages, to be in strife-filled relationships, to have lack in any area of life. He wants to restore all these areas. How can that be true? Because all good things pertaining to life (on this earth) and godliness in every area of our lives were provided by Jesus, from the Garden of Gethsemane to His Resurrection and Ascension. He is The Way out of every difficulty and every trial and He's our supply for every need, except one. We must be willing to suffer persecution for the sake of the gospel. What makes us willing? The fact that Jesus took every other problem for us and provided the solution. That's grace. Where is that grace when you need it? The Holy Spirit has all the answers to all the problems, and He's right there inside you.

So as a follower of Christ, be prepared for ridicule and humiliation. Be prepared for friends to turn against you, even some Christian friends, when you take a stand. And we may see the day when even in North America we suffer physical persecution as well, as many do in other areas of the world. But never again think that disease or lack in any area of life is within God's will for you as a New Covenant Christian.

Suffering as Job Did

You might ask, "But what about all Job's suffering? He went through pain and sickness, great sorrow and grief, devastating financial loss, and the destruction of his entire legacy.

Yes, he did, but everything is different now. You need to recognize these facts.

- Jesus is our role model now, not Job, so stop thinking the more we're like Job, the holier we are.
- Job lived under a different covenant than we have today. Our relationship with God is entirely different now than in Job's time. We have a better covenant based on better promises, and Job did not have the Holy Spirit.
- Job did, in a sense, bring calamity on himself. The first four verses of Job tell us he was a man of great integrity and great wealth, and he resisted evil in his life. But the fifth verse reveals that, though he worshipped the Lord, he didn't trust Him. He regularly made sacrifices, even for his adult children who didn't live under his roof, just in case they sinned. He lived in a state of fear. Job even admitted that what he had feared the most had befallen him. Fear is a magnet for calamity, because you are not trusting God.
- The Book of Job makes it sound as if Job's life was one long continuing series of tragedies, but in fact it was likely only about nine months. When you read Job, you'll notice that he mentions periods of weeks and of months, but not of years.
- There were a lot of erroneous beliefs revealed in Job and his friends, mostly centered around the lie of the enemy that Job's trials were chastisements from God. Scripture states in no uncertain terms that it was the devil attacking Job. Job said, "The Lord giveth and the Lord taketh away." No, God gives. It is satan that takes. The devil is the liar and thief and the bringer of disease and fear.
- God was bragging on Job! He told the devil he wasn't allowed to kill Job, but other than that, take his best shot, because God knew that Job would stand faithful. He knew Job would be a great example to us of deeply rooted reverence toward the Almighty. He would also show us an example of what not to do, and how not to react, though most Christians don't look at Job's story that way.
- Consider something you've probably never seen in Job before. The Lord revealed it to me just now, as I'm writing. The devil showed up in heaven uninvited, and God asked him where he'd come from. The devil answered that he'd been going to and fro upon the earth. (Why does the devil go to and fro on the earth according to scripture? To seek whom he may devour.) Then God said, "Have you considered Job?" God not only bragged on Job, He sicced the devil on him! Why would He do that to his faithful servant? The

devil was looking to **devour** somebody, to pour grief and illness and calamity on some poor soul, and God knew Job could take it and not lose faith. Any other man might have *cursed God and died*, as Job's wife suggested. It was Old Testament days, but even then, God healed His people. What Job suffered those nine months was not just illness, it was PERSECUTION from the devil. Job's suffering prevented another man from being utterly destroyed.

- There's always a good outcome with God if you wait for it, and there was for Job. It was far better than most of us know. We've all heard Job ended up with twice as much as he had before, but there's more, and I'll share it in the next book, since we're focusing on healing here.

The only thing that is ESSENTIAL to know about Job is that he was not under the covenant you are under today. You see, Jesus changed EVERYTHING. That's one of those words many Christians don't understand the meaning of. *Everything* means EVERYTHING. Had Job been born today, his dominion in Christ Jesus would have provided for Him to tell the devil where to go from the first moment of attack.

He's Calling Me Home

An old friend who was in the middle of a cancer scare once said to me, "You don't really believe in healing, do you? Don't you realize that when you get sick, it's God calling you home, and it's the sweetest call there is?" I was floored. Sweet or not, she had relief in her voice when she reported, "It's benign!"

I wish I'd had the guts back then to say, straight up, "If it's God's goodness to bring you home using disease, why are you hoping it's not cancerous?" If you believe that it's God's will that you have a disease so that you can go home soon, then what are you doing at the doctor's office scheduling tests and getting prescriptions? That would be disobedient. And if it's the ultimate kindness to have your Heavenly Father call you home, why are you asking for prayer?

> ...he has set his love upon Me, therefore I will deliver him; I will set him on high, because he has known My name. He shall call upon Me, and I will answer him; I will be with him in trouble; I will deliver him and honor him. With long life I will satisfy him, and show him My salvation."
> - Psalm 91:14-16 NKJV

God Always Chooses Life. Yes, Life Here on Earth

God wants to satisfy you with long life. Satisfy YOU. That sounds to me like YOU get to decide when you go! There are many examples in scripture of God recognizing our desire to live a long, full life, and He ensures us that this is His desire for us, too. After all, He created us as eternal beings on this earth — only through sin did death become the norm. God knows exactly how many days each of us will live because He doesn't operate in our time constraints. He *sees the end from the beginning*— but it is apparent that He made a way for us to participate in the determination of just how many days that will be.

> Honor thy father and thy mother: that thy days may be long upon the land that the LORD thy God giveth thee.
> - Exodus 20:12 KJV

> ...and that your days may be prolonged.
> - Deuteronomy 6:2 NKJV

> For I am hard-pressed between the two, having a desire to depart and be with Christ, which is far better. Nevertheless to remain in the flesh is more needful for you.
> - Philippians 1:23,24 NKJV

Paul couldn't decide which option he preferred — to go home to heaven, or to stay because the church needed him. This was not some daydream or a light-hearted conversation with a bro. He was writing a letter to the church at Philippi, in partnership with the Holy Spirit, which would later become part of the Bible. If it's in the Holy Bible, its inclusion was directed by God for a purpose — His purpose. Paul had no doubt that the choice he made would be honored by God. After all, He said He wanted US to be satisfied. We get to participate in the determination of how long our life will be!

If we're not raptured first, we are all going to die — but, by a long, drawn-out illness? You'll never find one verse of scripture indicating that is God's will for a single one of His children. And if it's not His will for you, why should you accept it? Death is God's enemy.

The Greek word thanatos refers primarily to death of the physical body.

> ...he would not see death before he had seen the Lord's Christ - Luke 2:26 NKJV

> Lord, I am ready to go with You, both to prison and to death - Luke 22:33 NKJV

> ...this sickness is not unto death - John 11:4 NKJV

> the Son of Man will be betrayed...and they will condemn Him to death - Matthew 20:18 NKJV

Note that Matthew 20:18 is referring to Jesus! So thanatos here is obviously referring to physical death, not being condemned to eternal separation from God.

Since God calls the death of our physical bodies an enemy, how can we think that God would put that on us? He could never employ the things of satan. No, anything that is God's enemy, we are supposed to war against.

> Yea, though I walk through the valley of the shadow of death, I shall fear no evil, for thou art with me...
> - Psalm 23:4 NKJV

Did King David say, "Yea, though You lead me to the valley of death"? No, the psalm says you're going THROUGH the valley of the shadow of death because He is with you, and because a shadow can't hurt you. He doesn't put the sickness on you. You're coming out the other side!

More proof?

> For I have no pleasure in the death of one who dies, says the Lord God, Therefore turn (repent) and live!
> - Ezekiel 18:32 NKJV

If God made you sick, He would essentially be a problem to be overcome. But the opposite is Truth — God is the answer to every problem.

> Inasmuch then as the children have partaken of the flesh and blood, He Himself likewise shared in the same, that through death He might destroy him who had the power of death, that is, the devil, and release those who through fear of death were all their lifetime subject to bondage.
> - Hebrews 2:14,15 NKJV

Jesus destroyed *the one who had the power of death, that is, the devil.* That's crystal clear — death is from the enemy, not from God. All sickness (satan trying to kill you) and death are your enemies.

God created perfection, masterpieces, each of us. Visit a nursing home, and what do you see? It is not perfection. It is the sad, ugly result of lies from the pit of hell, lifetimes of believing that sickness and aging are normal. They are not, not for believers. They are satan's perversion of God's perfection.

God is Saving Her from What's Ahead

This is not really a doctrine, more of an excuse for death, particularly of one who is young or has had a difficult life. It's on par with, "I guess God needed him in heaven." And it's bunk. I'm sorry, I know this is painful for some, but you have to get rid of these man-made expectations and excuses. They are things we say when somebody dies or is expected to. They are things we say when we don't know the truth. The problem is that these sayings further rob you, and others, of faith. When it looks hopeless, we think of reasons to justify death instead of thinking it's the perfect environment for God to show up and show off. Our culture is permeated by unbelief, and if you're going to make a difference in people's lives, including your own, you have to be in, but not OF this world, separate, a person set apart. (John 17:16; 1 Peter 2:9). Everything is possible in God, but we have to believe it and take it!

God provided healing two thousand years ago on the cross. He raised Jesus and others from the dead. Why would you think He can't heal somebody at the last moment? Why wouldn't you expect Him to smooth out the bumps in the road ahead for one who's trodden a rough path? He said He will be with us through every trial and tribulation and will deliver us out of them ALL.

> And the Lord will deliver me from every evil work and preserve me for His heavenly kingdom...
> - 2 Timothy 4:18 NKJV

> ...But God was with him and delivered him out of all his troubles, and gave him favor and wisdom...
> - Acts 7:9,10 NKJV

The enemy's passion is to lie, deceive, steal, kill and tear down. It's what he does. It's who he is. We have the tools to defend against his every ploy, but we have so much to learn about using them. Jesus will deliver you from every tribulation, but you first have to believe the scriptures that reveal that truth. Back in Isaiah, there's a scripture that does talk this about God taking people to save them from evil, but don't forget, that was Old Covenant, and Jesus changed everything.

We recently lost a person who sometimes went to our church and who was poverty-stricken and alcoholic. When he was taken ill and at death's door, most people prayed for God's will to be done because they don't know what you now know — that God's will is always to heal. Even the ones who believed God's will is to heal weren't certain in this case how to pray because this man had a hard life and by all indications would be healed only to face more of the same. They felt he'd be better off in heaven. News flash: we'd all be better off in heaven.

One friend prayed for the man's will to be done. She knew God would respect his wishes either way. (The way He had for my husband.)

But if God had His way, this kind man would have been healed and restored to a good, productive, bondage-free life, prospering in every area, because God is a God of restoration, and He supplies all our needs according to HIS riches. But this man had never heard any teaching that explained God's true will for him. We have to hear to believe and believe to receive.

God does not need us in heaven. He has work for us to do here on earth. Eternity is a very long time, and He is in no rush to have you join Him there.

We Are Jesus' Boots on the Ground

God does not take a person to heaven to keep them from facing something as bad or worse than their sickness. He wants to heal you then deliver you out of ALL your troubles! You are a chance for Him to show Himself strong and mighty. He IS your salvation.

Sometimes I wonder how sad God is that so many people don't read His Book, and those who do often don't grasp what it says. I frustrated Him for years, no doubt. I try not to anymore. It's a serious thing to not understand that the Bible means what it says. It's fortunate God loves us so much. Love really does cover a multitude of sins.

God Makes Us Ill for Unknown Reasons

> "And this woman, a daughter of Abraham as she is, whom Satan has bound for eighteen long years, should she not have been released from this bond on the Sabbath day?"
> - Luke 13:16 NASB

Who does it say bound her? It wasn't God. The scriptures do not equivocate. God does NOT make us sick or infirm. That is satan's workmanship.

> "The LORD will remove from you all sickness; and He will not put on you any of the harmful diseases of Egypt which you have known... - Deuteronomy 7:15 NASB

> For I will restore health to you, and your wounds I will heal, declares the LORD, - Jeremiah 30:17 ESV

There are so many proofs in the Bible to renew the mind of those who've been trapped in the teaching that God would actually harm us physically. He will not. Ever. For any reason.

> ...He himself took our infirmities and carried away our diseases. - Matthew 8:17 NASB

Why would He give you something that He suffered to take away from you? The scriptures tell us that He went through all that torture so that we don't have to suffer, even in this fallen world. It makes no sense to think that He'd turn right around and put those things back on us after that immeasurable pain. God is not schizophrenic. He is not going to do one thing and then the opposite, taking sides with satan.

> ...For what partnership has righteousness with lawlessness? Or what fellowship has light with darkness?
> - 2 Corinthians 6:14 ESV

> And if a house is divided against itself, that house Cannot stand. - Mark 3:25 NKJV

God says that His sheep know His voice. He is the GOOD Shepherd. A good shepherd would never beat his sheep. Psalm 23 says, "Thy rod and thy staff, they comfort me." Yet many think they are tools of punishment or at least discipline. They are not. Real life shepherds will tell you — the staff is to guide, to rescue, to safely pull you up when you fall. The rod is not to beat the sheep — it's for beating off the wolves!

God Hurts Us so He can Show Off Later

Some see the John 9 account of the man born blind as stating that God causes disease or physical infirmity so that He can show off at the right time and heal it. This is so far from the truth. First and foremost, scripture tells us over and over that God heals His children, not that He harms us. We also know that He does not contradict Himself. It's even impossible for Him to do. So when we see a scripture passage that seems to contradict what the Bible tells us is God's character, then we know that it's because of our misunderstanding or something lost in translation, not because God is schizo. This is a prime example of making a doctrine from one verse of the Bible, even though it sounds as if it counters what the rest of the scriptures prove about the Father's nature and character. Now consider these points about John 9:

- There were multitudes (uncountable numbers) of people to heal and no doubt numerous were blind from birth. Why would God make one particular person blind when the devil had already supplied plenty for Him to heal?
- If God made people sick, why would Jesus be healing everyone? A house divided against itself cannot stand (Matthew 12:25).
- By the same logic, did Jesus go around making some people sick while He was here? Of course not. But if it was God's will that some people were sick for ANY reason, then Jesus would have done some imparting of illness, because He was here to execute God's will. (And if that were the case, how many people do you think would have taken the chance of being ministered to?)
- Jesus established in John 9:3-5 that sin (by the man or his parents) had nothing to do with the man's birth defect, and that He was going to heal him and as many people as possible while He was on earth, for God's glory and to authenticate the gospel.

Now for historical context. Only this one time is it recorded that Jesus made mud and put it on the man's face. This suggests, because we were formed from the earth, that the man was born without eyes, so Jesus was using the earth to form the eyes. My understanding is that the Jews of the time believed that only the Messiah would be able to do these two things:

heal someone blind from birth and cleanse the lepers. As history records, Jesus did both.

The wording as translated makes this difficult to see at first, but if you read all of Jesus' words in that encounter, you will see that the context is about timing, accomplishing as much as possible while He was still present on earth. The man was not singled out by God to be born blind so that in God's perfect timing he could be used to display God's abilities; that man just happened to be the blind one that was in the right place at the right time to receive!

> ... "It was not that this man sinned, or his parents, but that the works of God might be displayed in him. We must work the works of him who sent me while it is day; night is coming, when no one can work. As long as I am in the world, I am the light of the world." - John 9:3-5 ESV

But that the works of God might be displayed in him is just another example of God making what the devil had meant for evil turn and bite him in the backside.

Does God cause calamity, in this case a birth defect, as a way to later turn the person toward Himself? I heard Audrey Mack (https://www.*gotellministry.org*) in November of 2019 answer that. She said that's like suspecting the paramedics of causing a traffic accident. Isn't that a great analogy?

God is your first responder! Nobody is faster on the scene than He is with all the rescue equipment at hand. But He didn't cause the accident. In fact, He tried to help you avoid it. Were you not paying attention?

> Only — goodness and kindness pursue me, All the days of my life... - Psalm 23:6 YLT

God's Love Makes You FEARLESS

God says your body is the temple where His Holy Spirit resides — the third part of our Triune God actually lives inside you if you are saved. Would God defile His own temple? And how could He employ the devil's tactics? It will never happen. He is INFINITE. He has infinite numbers of ways to lead, guide and direct you that do not include something we'd jail any earthly parent for doing to their child. We don't need God in order to get sick or have accidents. The devil has set up an environment in which we can do all that on our own. And on our own, we WILL do exactly that.

God's perfect love casts out fear (1 John 4:18). How could that be true if God was the one harming you?

Over and over the Word proves to us that God wants us for his own — "that none should perish" (2 Peter 3:9). Saved yet or not, He wants to continually draw you nearer and nearer to Him in relationship. Scripture tells us it's His goodness that draws you. You are not drawn by the thought that He'll soon show you His love and His desire to make you more like Jesus through bodily harm. That's twisted, devil-inspired thinking. (Jesus was never sick, by the way, so being more like Jesus includes walking in divine health.) What kind of parent would God be if He actually made you sick or broke your bones? Abusive and to be feared in the modern usage of the word.

> ...Yes, I have loved you with an everlasting love, therefore with lovingkindness have I drawn you and continued My faithfulness to you. - Jeremiah 31:3 AMPC

Such a beautiful scripture, a beautiful picture in words of His ongoing tender care for you. How could anyone read this, then think that He could intentionally hurt you? Scripture tells you that Jesus is faithful to you even when you forsake Him. You are loved with *an everlasting love*!

Satan Has No Power Over My Body

Glad to hear it. But then, please explain to me why you're sick. The Gospels clearly state that sickness and disease are the works of the enemy.

> ...how God anointed Jesus of Nazareth with the Holy Spirit and power, and how he went around doing good and **healing all who were under the power of the devil**, because God was with him. - Acts 10:38 NIV

So if there is sickness of any kind in your body, the enemy is exerting power over you. I'm not saying he has the authority to. If you're saved, he has no authority to attack you. But since when did a thief or killer ask permission to steal or murder? He doesn't wait for permission; he waits for an opportunity to sneak in and will stay until either you tell him to go or you're dead, whichever comes first. He's doing it without authority because you haven't stopped him, because he roams about looking for whom he MAY devour (1 Peter 5:8).

"Mmmmm.... He looks yummy. I can have him with a side of cancelled mission trip and loss of faith for dessert!"

Tell the devil you're off the menu! Put your foot down and say, "NO!" We're going to put a stop to his mischief, you and I, because Jesus has taken all authority back from the enemy, and given us His power and authority to use. The enemy is already defeated. Jesus won the war! All we have to do is sweep up behind Him, take out the trash, mop up, evict the trespassers.

We live in a fallen world, meaning that the world is in a state of atrophy and decay. This state affects the earth and everything in it. The effects on our physical bodies include aging, acute and chronic illnesses, and death. All this stems from the entrance of sin into the world. So up to now, perhaps not realizing that your health problems are from the enemy, how have you been dealing with this state of atrophy? I would assume by eating right, exercising, and taking either natural or modern medicine. I truly hope that's going well. But what about when it doesn't?

Here's something you probably haven't thought about. You know all those multitudes Jesus healed while He was here in bodily form? Every single one of them was on the Mediterranean diet! Sooner or later nearly everyone needs to be healed of something.

> **If You Can Say "NO" to Sin, You Can Say "NO" to Sickness**

Regardless of whether or not you trust the medical system or whether or not you trust nature, if you are not relying on God, you are relying on self-effort and leaning on the wisdom of man. Yes, you can say that God put those things here for us. And, by all means if God tells you to have surgery (I have) or take certain medicines or supplements (I do), absolutely you should. And by all means pray over your medicines, supplements, vaccines, food and exercises. Bless them to do only good in your body. Stand on the scripture that states nothing poisonous will hurt you (Mark 16:18) when you're taking medications or eating. Trusting Him fully is what God wants from you. It's what He wants you to grow into. It's what I'm hoping to grow into.

This is part of the reason we receive healing in different ways at different times. Your beliefs change depending on who or what you're reading or listening to, whether or not you've been renewing your mind, and on your experiences. The more time we spend with the Lord and in the Word, the more our minds are renewed, the more we trust Him, and the more expectation we have to receive from Him because we better know that His nature is to give and to heal.

Know this: if you're operating on your own in this world in the area of health, you're fighting an uphill battle. Sooner or later, the fallen nature of our world will impact your physical body. Perhaps it already has, and you've relied only on doctors. Whenever that time comes, you really have only two choices, because there are only two teams on the field. Decide which team you want to be on.

> ...Asa developed a disease in his feet, and his disease became increasingly severe. Yet even in his disease **he didn't seek the Lord but only the physicians**. Asa rested with his fathers; he died in the forty-first year of his reign.
> - 2 Chronicles 16:12,13 CSB

> A woman suffering from bleeding for twelve years, who had spent all she had on doctors and yet could not be healed by any, approached from behind and touched the end of his robe. Instantly her bleeding stopped.
> - Luke 8:43,44 CSB

You can agree with God's report, and follow what the Word says and what the Holy Spirit's strategy is for your healing. He will meet you at your point of faith, and that may even include some of man's methods. **Speak only faith;** rest in the knowledge that Jesus healed you at the whipping post and that you are now learning to receive that healing.

Or you can agree with the enemy (which involves believing the doctors' reports instead of what the Word says about you) and allow the agents of death to drag you in that direction. Blessing or curse? Life or death? It's your decision. Not deciding is a decision for man's wisdom, and we know which team that is really a decision for.

If you're a believer and want to live the abundant life you've been promised, then you need to take God at His word. You need to recognize that the pain, the cancer, the diabetes, the allergies or whatever the problem is in your body, big or small, is from the devil who comes to kill, steal and destroy and should be eliminated from your life. You are greatly loved. Do not allow the deceiver to convince you that God isn't interested in your physical body. **He created it.**

The devil can only have power over you if YOU allow it. It is often not an easy fight, but it's one you're in whether you want to be or not. So fight the good fight of faith. As a New Covenant believer, you have the authority to evict the enemy and his works from your body.

CHAPTER 13
He's Able but Is He Willing?

Questioning God's Intent Toward You

We all likely agree on the fact that God CAN heal. He's all-powerful. He can do anything and everything. But will He? Does He want to? And when will He get around to it? Jesus told us that if you've seen Him, You've seen the Father. How was this truth lived out in Jesus' ministry here on Earth, and what does it have to do with healing today? He tells us in John 14:10 & 31, among other scriptures, that He did only what the Father told Him to do and said only what the Father told Him to say.

> Jesus' Attitude Toward Healing Is the Father's Attitude Toward Healing

So then, what was the Father's attitude toward healing? What did Jesus do, at the Father's direction, for everyone that needed healing? He healed them. He healed them all. Right then.

> Jesus was going about all Galilee teaching in their synagogues, and proclaiming the good news of the reign, and healing every disease, and every malady among the people and his fame went forth to all Syria, and they brought to him all having ailments, pressed with manifold sicknesses and pains, and demoniacs, and lunatics and paralytics, and he healed them. - Matthew 4:23,24 YLT

When you read in the gospels about Jesus' healing ministry, note how many inclusive words — *all* and *every* and *them* — are used to describe His acts.

> But the multitudes perceiving it followed him; and he welcomed them, and spake to them of the kingdom of God, and them that had need of healing he cured.
> - Luke 9:11 ASV

> He forgives all my sins and heals all my diseases.
> - Psalm 103:3 NLT

As a Christian you know that God's will is the driving force behind every good thing that happens on this earth (James 1:17). The Bible tells us that Jesus performed so many miracles that the world couldn't contain all the books it would take to write about them (John 21:25). That tells me that the signs (attesting miracles) the Holy Spirit did cause to be recorded in scripture are there for specific reasons. There are lessons to be gleaned from each one, truths to be discerned.

Scripture records (Matthew 8:2, Luke 5:12) that a leper asked Jesus point blank one day if He was willing to heal him. Jesus replied, "I am willing." After the multitude of healings Jesus had already performed, you would think *are you willing* would be an unnecessary question. But God put it in the Bible just for you, because you've asked that question in your heart, haven't you? I know I have. Jesus touched the leper and healed him. Why is that noteworthy?

It was against Jewish law to touch a leper. Doing so made you unclean and an outcast, as the leper was unclean. That's a little easier for us to understand since social distancing came into being. In that world system, the unclean defiles the clean, the unholy blemishes the holy. But God makes the unclean clean with a touch, makes the unholy holy, and makes the unworthy worthy. And He does that for you and me.

Another exhilarating revelation is that in the original Greek, *thelo*, the word translated as *willing* or *I will*, has much more depth than in English. What Jesus said is more like, "I will delight in doing it; It is my constant desire; and It is my very nature to do this for you." He is so wonderful.

If you believe that it's not always God's will to heal, please, show me New Testament scripture to back up your assertion. Everybody who needed healing was healed. Period. He never turned anyone away or even told them to be patient. He delighted in healing. And remember, Jesus only did what our Father told Him to do and only said what our Father told Him to say.

If God Wants Me healed, He'll Heal Me

That's what my pastor-friend believed, and now there's another widow and two more fatherless children on this earth. Such sadness is never God's will. Wondering IF God wants you well is one of the easiest traps for Christians to fall into. It's also a slap in the face of the One Who loves you most. That's your first mistake. Your second is thinking you have no part to play due to God's sovereignty.

> Yea, they turned back and tempted God, and **LIMITED** the Holy One of Israel. - Psalm 78:41 NKJV

How do we limit God? Through our unbelief and our unscriptural speech — our idle words. (When you're ready to hear it, you can substitute the word *YOU/YOURS* for every *WE/OUR* in those sentences.) God wants you healed more than you want to be well. He loves you with every fiber of His being. That's why He healed you two thousand years ago. But YOU have to choose it and implement it. If you think you can lay in that bed just hoping that you'll wake up healed one morning, then one morning you just won't wake up.

At creation God gave us dominion over the earth, and He gave us free will. He limited His sovereignty on this earth when He gave these amazing gifts. But then we gave our dominion to satan. What does that mean in our everyday lives? Sickness, all manner of sins, anxiety, the work week, financial strain, malnutrition, relationship problems, rebellion, aging, unrest, wars, mental disorders, stress, worry, idolatry in every form imaginable, pesticides, doubt and unbelief toward God, lack of peace, drugs with side effects, corporate and personal greed, abortion, all types of temptations, crumbling family structure, trials and tribulation, addiction, death. Everything bad in this world is a result of the Fall of Man from his position of sonship at creation.

But Jesus restored you to the Father! So when you use your God-given free will to choose Jesus as your Lord and Savior, you can become a son. Not a servant, a New Covenant son or daughter. You are a king and a priest. And what are you to do with this unearned status? Join the family business, which is to pick that dominion back up and use it to destroy the works of the devil. That is what Jesus did while He was here, and that is what you're to do now. **One of those evil works is the illness in your body.**

God has told YOU to fight the enemy. YOU are to invite the Holy Spirit to provide the power you need to accomplish God's will on this earth. YOU are to pray, asking of your own free will for God to intervene in earthly matters. YOU are to use the authority Jesus left with YOU. YOU are to use His Name. YOU are to study His Word in order to know His will and act accordingly. YOU are to don the whole armor of God. YOU are to resist the devil until he flees from YOU. YOU are to pray to gain discernment, wisdom, and knowledge.

God already did His part by providing everything you will ever need. He sent Jesus, our Redeemer, Who defeated the enemy, Who paid for your *SOZO* salvation, Who left you His own shalom peace, and then He sent the Holy Spirit with supernatural knowledge and power to help you.

Responsibility — I know this may not be what you want to hear. It's not what I wanted to hear. Don't think I didn't whine for days, "But I don't want to do all that. I want You to do it for me! It's so much easier for you!" On the other hand, it's empowering! And, it explains a lot. Jesus won the war for us and went back to Heaven, and we're to enforce His victory.

> For His divine power has bestowed upon us all things that [are requisite and suited] to life (**zoe**) and godliness, through the [full, personal] knowledge of Him Who called us by *and* to His own glory and excellence (virtue).
> - 2 Peter 1:3 AMPC

This is the provision for walking in God's blessings, promises, and commandments. You already have everything you need to be healed and walk in divine health from now on — everything and more. It doesn't matter if you don't FEEL that you have all that, you do because God's Word is true. How did He give it to us? You got it when you accepted Christ, and the Holy Spirit came to live inside you!

Most of your past prayers were useless if you were begging God for something He's already given you. So when you were prostrate, praying for healing, God was trying to tell you He's already provided it, and now it's up to you to allow it to manifest in your life. More good news is that it's much easier to release something God's already put inside you than it is to storm heaven's gates trying to get God to give you something when He's already done it. (What are you doing outside the gates, anyway?)

Now YOU fight the devil. YOU believe. YOU send your faith out on the playing field, and don't let it back on the bench until you have what you desire, whether it takes five seconds or five years. YOU ask the Holy Spirit to go out into your flesh and quicken your mortal body. YOU lay hold of healing, and never let go. YOU start taking God at His word. YOU change the way you talk. YOU start limiting the world's influence on your mind. YOU start focusing on Jesus instead of the doctor's report. YOU start praising God, remembering everything He's done in your life. YOU start taking the Word as if it's your medicine. YOU resist the devil until he flees from YOU. You have many weapons in your arsenal, and YOU have to use them. That's the way God set the system up. It's the responsibility that comes with free will, dominion, and authority.

Paul's Thorn

> Messenger = Angel
> Messenger of Satan = Demon

For decades, perhaps even centuries, it's been taught from the pulpit that the infamous thorn in Paul's side was a physical ailment — in First Baptist, I heard it was a crippled leg. Since then I've heard that the most popular malady is an oozing eye disease, ophthalmia. How is it that we and our spiritual leaders have been so deceived for so long? The scripture is very clear on the matter. Let's see what the Word actually says about Paul, in Paul's own words.

> And lest I should be exalted above measure by the abundance of the revelations, a thorn in the flesh was given to me, the messenger of Satan to buffet me, lest I be exalted above measure. - 2 Corinthians 12: 7 NKJV

So it's obvious that what Paul called a *thorn in the flesh*, or in some translations, a *thorn in the side*, was a MESSENGER OF SATAN — an evil spirit or demon. It went ahead of Paul in his travels and stirred up people against him — "we wrestle not against flesh and blood..." (Ephesians 6:12). This is clearly evidenced by the floggings, imprisonment, and other persecutions, including being stoned to death (from which Paul was immediately raised, God's grace being sufficient).

Don't believe me? That's what interlinear concordances were made for. The original Greek word translated *messenger* is *aggelos*. It's used 186 times in the KJV, seven times as *messenger* (*def.* one who is sent) and 179 times as *angel*. Never once does *Strong's Concordance* define it as anything other than a personality. Why, for this one, single verse, have we altered the definition to *a grievous malady*? That's some serious deception — just think about how we've been brainwashed for generations with this one lie. That one verse, when we buy into the deception, would mean that Jesus didn't accomplish healing with the stripes Isaiah and Peter tell us of. We have bought that story, even though the disciples *healed them all* (Acts 5:15), and many others healed according to the scriptures. And if Paul was not healthy and quite fit, how could he ever survive the prisons and the physical persecution that he went through?

That one altered definition, my friend, is a prime example of the wisdom of man and the perversion of God's word by the enemy. An *aggelos* is a spirit being. So why did Paul describe it as a *thorn in the flesh*? It's a

Hebrewism. A *thorn in the flesh* is the same thing as a pain in the um...backside.

> But if you do not drive out the inhabitants of the land from before you, then it shall be that those whom you let remain *shall be* irritants in your eyes and **thorns in your sides**, and they shall harass you in the land where you dwell.
> - Numbers 33:55 NKJV

> And there shall no longer be a pricking brier or a **painful thorn** for the house of Israel from among all who are around them, who despise them. Then they shall know that I am the Lord God. - Ezekiel 28:24 NKJV

The thorn has nothing to do with physical infirmity — it is a person or people group that harasses, just like Paul's harassing demon. God answered Paul's prayer by stating that His grace was sufficient, and proceeded to rescue Paul out of every situation this evil messenger inspired.

I wonder if this verse, with its *thorns in your eyes* might be where the idea of Paul having ophthalmia first started?

> ...they will become snares and traps for you, whips on your backs and **thorns in your eyes**, - Joshua 23:13 NIV

Believers knew they could touch Paul's clothing and be healed the same as with Jesus. That was initiated by the woman with the issue of blood. (I'm looking forward to meeting that brave, bold woman of God one day.) We also know that Paul put cloths against his body and then cut them up into smaller handkerchiefs which were dispatched to believers all over the region as a point of faith for healing (Acts 19:12). From a practical perspective, we should consider that ophthalmia is quite contagious. The cloths carried the healing power of God to the recipients, not a contagion. Who would have wanted anything off Paul's body if he had pus oozing from his eyes, constantly having to wipe them, probably with those very handkerchiefs! That's just gross.

Why didn't God just zap the evil spirit and save Paul the physical pain of the whippings and stoning he endured? We're talking about persecution here, not illness, and that's the one thing we're called to suffer. You may recall hearing that in times of persecution, the church grows, and that is more important than anyone's comfort or life, because of the eternal consequences for others.

> ...So for the sake of Christ, I am well pleased and take pleasure in infirmities, insults, hardships, persecutions, perplexities and distresses; for when I am weak [in human strength], then am I [truly] strong (able, powerful in divine strength). - 2 Corinthians 12:10 AMPC

Nowhere in scripture will you find an ill, diseased, or crippled disciple. (We'll deal with Timothy in a moment.) They were whipped, exhausted, beheaded, crucified and otherwise persecuted FOR HIS NAME'S SAKE. But they never died of disease. Why then should you? You shouldn't, and *you* don't have to if you believe as Paul believed, in the gospel of grace.

> But I do not account my life of any value nor as precious to myself, if only I may finish my course and the ministry that I received from the Lord Jesus, to testify to the gospel of the grace of God. - Acts 20:24 ESV

> For I am not ashamed of the gospel, for it is the power of God for salvation to everyone who believes, to the Jew first and also to the Greek. - Romans 1:16 ESV

God Didn't Heal Timothy

Christians will bring up "Timothy's frequent infirmities" as proof that God's will is not always to heal. I cry, "Foul." This is one of the most misunderstood passages of scripture ever.

> No longer drink only water, but use a little wine for your stomach's sake and your frequent infirmities.
> - 1 Timothy 5:23 NKJV

First we're going to look at *Timothy's frequent infirmities* the two ways most of us have been taught to understand it.

1. Timothy had digestive issues, so Paul told him to drink some wine each day for his stomach. People take this to mean either that
Wine is good for our stomachs so we should drink some every day, or
because they believe drinking is a sin, they believe Paul obviously meant grape juice — new wine.

Rebuttal: What some Christians quote as permission to drink alcohol is actually referring to the use of wine as an astringent or antiseptic, to drink wine or add wine to his water to reduce the risk of becoming ill from the local well. Contaminated water was a common problem. And no, grape juice would not be the least bit helpful in this respect — Paul said wine and meant wine.

2. Timothy had digestive issues, so it's obviously not always God's will to heal or He would have healed Timothy.

Rebuttal: If it were not the will of God for Timothy to be well, then Paul's advice would have countered the will of God. This scripture does NOT lend credence to the idea that God's will is not always for healing, because Paul's intent is obviously for Timothy to be free of this discomfort. Paul would have told Timothy to man up and live with the symptoms if Paul believed it was God's will for Timothy to be ill. He would have admonished Timothy to find the spiritual lesson God was trying to impart, to be a shining example to all the other sick Christians, to show his patience in this trial, or some other holy sounding instruction. No, Paul gave him practical advice on how to avoid the problem going forward. Therefore, Paul obviously believed God's will was for the healthy functioning of Timothy's body.

So, neither of those two understandings of Timothy's "infirmities" is correct. Furthermore, think about this.

> "And ye shall serve the LORD your God, and he shall bless thy bread, and thy water; and I will take sickness away from the midst of thee." - Exodus 23:25 KJV

These men knew the Torah. They knew their food and drink was blessed by God, so there was no illness from it. But let's say that their food wasn't blessed. No problem. They would have taken authority, cleansed the water, and cursed the pathogens— problem dealt with. But again, let's just say no authority was used. Simple — Paul would have healed Timothy. Our brains have trouble accepting that standing on scripture, taking authority and prayer work every time. We've been taught the opposite. We don't mix our words or God's with faith. But Paul and Timothy had no such issue.

So how could there have been an illness that made it needful to take wine? The "fact" that Timothy was ill at all goes against the nature and character of God and His Word, which Timothy and Paul operated in.

The scripture from Exodus says, "ye shall serve the Lord." So it's a conditional promise, or was in the times of Exodus. Raise your hand if you think Paul and Timothy were serving God. Raise your other hand if you know we have a better Covenant with better promises now than when Exodus was written. You're now in the perfect position to thank God for revealing the truth I'm about to share, because we've been reading this passage of scripture all wrong for generations!

This is straight from God — I've never heard anyone teach this, and I listen to a variety of teachings most every day. Had I not renewed my mind to the fact that God's will is always for health and life, I would not have been able to receive this revelation. He will reveal truth to you, too, when you pursue it from the depth of your heart.

So here's the thing: Timothy wasn't sick at all! In that part of the world adding wine to water was a normal practice, so why would Timothy need to be told to do that? This verse is not even about physical ailments. It's a parable, or perhaps due to its simplicity, a better term would be illustration or metaphor. Remember that I said "context is everything?" This passage is a classic example. Read verses 22 and 24 together:

> Do not lay hands on anyone hastily, nor share in other people's sins; keep yourself pure...Some men's sins are clearly evident, preceding them to judgement, but those of some men follow later. - 1 Timothy 5:22,24 NKJV

It makes perfect sense now, and it's easy to follow. Many have taught that this refers to laying hands on when ministering healing, but if that was the case, the Bible would be lying when it said in Luke 10:19, "you will in no way be harmed" when you lay hands on the sick or cast out demons. Paul is advising Timothy about sending others out into ministry — impartation and ordination. He's saying to be careful of who you commission under your spiritual headship — be certain of that person's morality and integrity because they're carrying your name, and their actions will reflect on you and your ministry. So there's our context. Now, add verse 23 back in.

> v22 - Do not lay hands on anyone hastily, nor share in other people's sins; keep yourself pure.
> v23 - No longer drink only water, but use a little wine for your stomach's sake and your frequent infirmities.
> v24 - Some men's sins are clearly evident, preceding them to judgement, but those of some men follow later.

Why, in a letter instructing on ordination, interrupt the lesson with a mention of the addressee's tummy trouble? There's a complete lack of cohesiveness if verse 23 is taken literally. But if you see that it's a real-life metaphor for what Paul is trying to convey, suddenly there's clarity.

Paul uses what to them is a common occurrence — organisms living in their drinking water — to illustrate his point. These organisms make the water impure, but you cannot see them, so the water's offensiveness is not revealed until later when your belly begins to ache. Suddenly verse 23 makes complete sense in that cultural and historic context.

Well-intentioned people may come to you wanting to be part of your ministry. In some, it's easy to see by the sin in their lives that they are not ready for ministry yet, so you don't even consider sending them out. The water is murky, so you're not going to drink it. Other people look like they're ready — they love people, appear to live a godly life, are eager to serve. The water looks crystal clear. But never make a hasty decision, because sin is not always so obvious. Pathogens may be lurking in the water, and soon you'll suffer from its corruption. You can be duped by the enemy into sending out people who do more harm than good. As they gain influence and prestige in the eyes of others, corruption surfaces. (I'm sure a few names come to mind.) Paul's message to Timothy is about choosing who to send into the mission field, and he illustrates it with a commonly understood practice.

Here's a modern example of the same type of metaphor.

> "University education is so expensive these days, and graduates are a dime a dozen in the job market — 'Want fries with that?' I'm considering steering my kid toward the trades. They're always in demand and much less costly to qualify for."

This revelatory experience with God really drove home for me how important it is to know His character in order to comprehend the meaning of God's Word. But no matter how we look at verse 23, it most definitely does not indicate that God's will is in question regarding healing.

I Brought This on Myself

You might say, "I've been (smoking or drinking or eating sweets or working with pesticides, etc.) for years, and I knew better! I brought this on myself." Ok, so you believe you deserve the problems you get yourself into, and God won't do anything about those issues? So many of us believe that way. Whether we verbalize it or not, it's deep in our psyches. I know it has been in mine, and I still do battle with it. Let's see what the Bible says.

> Fools because of their transgression, and because of their iniquities, are afflicted. Then they cry unto the Lord in their trouble, and he saveth them out of their distresses. He sent his word, and healed them, and delivered them from their destructions. Oh that men would praise the Lord for his goodness, and for his wonderful works to the children of men! - Psalm 107:17, 19-21 KJV

Matthew 1:1-16 expounds on the genealogy of Jesus. At the time these scriptures were written, it was highly unusual to enter the names of women in a list of ancestors. But in Jesus' lineage, four women made the cut. Is Mary, His mother, one of them? No. What about Sara, wife of Abraham, Father of the Faith? No, she's not listed. How about Leah who represents the law or Rachel who represents grace? Nope. The women listed in the Bible as ancestors in direct line to our Lord and Savior Jesus Christ are Tamar, Rahab, Ruth and Bathsheba. He could have mentioned myriad women known for faith, love, even holiness. But He chose instead to illustrate His grace to us.

Tamar slept with her father-in-law through deception and prostitution in order to bear children. Rahab was an Amorite (from a heathen nation) and a prostitute in Jericho. Ruth was a good woman, but a Moabite — an unclean gentile from a nationality specifically prohibited any benefits by the Jewish law of that day. And Bathsheba, well, she's the icing on the cake, isn't she? Sleeping with King David before and after he had her husband murdered tells us a lot about her. And bathing on the rooftop? She must have known David would see her from the palace terraces.

The Most High God lined these women up to be the forebears of His very own Son! Why would He do that? Why not use men and women we could consider righteous, and upright to be the ancestors of the Savior? What was God thinking?

He's showing us that His grace covers all our situations and sin: sins of omission – including iniquity, being born with a sin nature, represented by Ruth the Moabite; and sins of commission creating the mess we live in by our own bad decisions and actions, hurting others and ourselves. Yet God rescued each of them and drew attention to them by listing them in Jesus' genealogy.

Tamar bore twin sons — one, Perez, became King of Persia and was the great-great-great-grandfather of Salmon. Rahab and her family were the only survivors of Jericho. She married this same Salmon, a mighty warrior of the Israelite army as they were taking the Promised Land. She gave birth to Boaz. Ruth went from abject poverty to the wife of Boaz, a wealthy landowner and man of great integrity. In fact, Ruth and Boaz's story is a picture of Jesus as the Kinsman-Redeemer, one of the names of Christ based on the marriage traditions of the time. (Ruth represents the church, the Bride of Christ.) Ruth and Boaz were grandparents to David, who Israel still considers its greatest king. Bathsheba married David, and one of their sons was Solomon, the world's wisest and richest king ever to live. We could consider three of these women the worst of the worst, yet they were highly blessed and favored by God

Can you imagine any greater blessing than having the Son of God in your lineage? It is impossible to earn that great honor. These women were singled out for our attention because of their **shortcomings**. Some committed sins so great as to warrant a death sentence in earthly courts of the day, yet they were used by the Almighty to be our examples. How can that be? Because they're not examples in their own worth. They're examples of how God's grace covers all our sin, shame, and weaknesses and makes us blessed and highly favored in spite of how short of the mark of His excellence we fall.

What does this have to do with healing health problems you feel you brought on yourself? If you're born again, Jesus saved you from the consequences of your sins—your sin was remitted. Where did those sins of commission come from? Did they fall from the sky? Did somebody else put them on you? No. YOU committed them. Yet Jesus redeemed you. He paid for those sins, even though you brought every single one of them on yourself. These four women illustrate that when you have been redeemed, God sees you completely restored to His perfection. If He didn't, how could He have made these women Jesus' forebears?

Healing is the same as forgiveness. It doesn't matter if you brought it on yourself, the healing is still there, waiting for you, paid for. It was paid for while you were still an enemy of God. You have been redeemed out of the messes of your own making, whether that mess is sin, broken relationships, lack, or poor health.

You are blessed and highly favored, deeply loved, and covered by God's grace and Jesus' blood. Be healed, just as you are forgiven.

It Isn't Always His Will to Heal

Yes, it is — always, every time, no matter what. In the previous chapters I've alluded to this, but I'm going to be more specific now to make sure you get this cemented in your mind. Here is the next step, the next truth, beyond healing being God's will.

Healing is ALWAYS God's will. That's a very bold statement, and it's true. Physical healing here on this earth and right now is ALWAYS God's will for you, your loved ones, every person on this earth. How can I state that without doubt? Three simple reasons:

1. Because He created our bodies to heal themselves. When you scratch your arm, in a few days it has healed. Cells throughout our body reproduce themselves constantly. Skin knows how to make skin, the liver regenerates, bones mend, lungs clear themselves. If you have the right fuel (nutrition) and are not completely overloaded with toxins, your body will prevent disease from taking hold, will heal itself when a sickness gets past your defenses, and repair any wounds you sustain. That's how God designed you. If He designed you and created you to remain healthy, why would you think your health is not His will?

2. Because even when we ourselves let satan into the garden, permitting him to bring in sin, sickness and death (this fallen world), God came back to earth as Jesus to make a way to get us out of the predicament we'd gotten ourselves into. Two thousand years ago He came back and took that cat-o'-nine-tails so that you could once again live in divine health, and you're wasting His pain. But as you come to understand what Jesus accomplished by that scourging, you need to also understand that He's not going to come back for more lashes every time somebody wants healing. He did it once, for all people, for all time. His will is that none should perish, and that's just as true for your physical life as it is for eternal life. He did it all at Calvary. It has been (past tense) accomplished. You were healed by his stripes.

3. Because as we've already established, sin and sickness are enmeshed and come only from the enemy. If you believe that God doesn't always heal, how can you believe that He always forgives? If you believe God's will is for none to perish but for all to be forgiven and spend eternity in Heaven, which the Bible makes very clear, then you must also believe that it is God's will to heal all based on the scriptural proofs we've already covered. Otherwise, He would be destroying the work of the devil in one case and not the next. God wants EVERY evil work crushed.

And there it is, folks, the answer many of you are looking for. You don't have to call God down and convince Him to heal you, which is what most of our prayers have been striving after. It's already done. It's already paid for. It's been delivered right to your door. It's what He planned for you from the beginning.

Have you ever noticed that we make excuses for God? And by this, I mean, as opposed to excuses for ourselves. We don't say, "I couldn't maintain my faith. I gave up. So I'm believing a lie somewhere, and need to learn more." Or, "I messed up and started believing the doctor above God." Instead we say, "This faith stuff doesn't work. God may heal some people, but not me." Or, "Don't listen to those faith preachers; they're straight from the devil. All they want is your money."

Past Failure Is No Excuse for Inaction Today

I'm here to tell you, God's grace is all you will ever need. You don't even really need faith (see Chapter 31). You get to share in the divine nature, because you are covered with His blood.

> His divine power has given us everything required for life (zoe) and godliness through the knowledge of him who called us by his own glory and goodness. By these he has given us very great and precious promises, so that through them you may share in the divine nature, escaping the corruption (destruction, perishing, death) that is in the world because of evil desire.
> - 2 Peter 1:3,4 CSB

Corruption here doesn't mean the kind of corruption in Chicago politics. The Greek word translated *corruption* here is the same word used for the corruptible body in 1 Corinthians 15:53,54. And what did you learn *zoe* means? Physical and abundant life here on earth. So stop blaming God that you're not healed. Instead, figure out what YOU are believing wrong, and start believing right. I lost my husband. Trust me in this: past failure is no excuse for not believing. Instead, make it your motivation to learn more, trust more, and believe correctly.

CHAPTER 14
He's Willing but Is He Able?

It Runs in the Family

My mother and grandmother have/had thyroid issues. I had allergies and my son has allergies (but not for much longer). My dad went into anaphylactic shock due to a penicillin injection, and my maternal grandfather was also allergic to it, so my brother and I have never taken it — just common sense. We all have genetic weak spots in this fallen world.

Genetic Tendencies

Let me make something completely clear: it does not matter whether your physical problem is a mole in the same place your dad had one or breast cancer that has taken three generations of women in your family. Healing has been provided and is yours for the taking. Headache? Healed. Goiter? Healed. The plague? Healed. MS? Healed. To God it doesn't matter how minor or major your problem is, whether it's inherited or contagious, from an injury or completely spiritual in nature. Healed. Nothing is more difficult to heal just because it's been passed down through the family line. It's done. Jesus never asked anyone if their infirmity was genetic or whether they'd fallen trying to jump from one housetop to another in a juvenile stunt. Healed. It does not matter how many generations your family has had this problem. It didn't come from God, and it's no more difficult to heal than a cold your kids brought home from school. Done.

Generational Curses

Are these genetic tendencies what people call generational curses? I guess it depends on what you've been taught about generational curses. Some people have never heard of them; some have searched their family histories back to the Druids to find some clue as to problems they're dealing with now. Alcoholism may run in a family, high blood pressure, colon cancer, bad tempers, allergies or criminality. In reality, it's either genetics or the choices made in this fallen world — nature or nurture. Either way, it doesn't matter.

Let me state emphatically — if you are saved, you are not subject to any curse of any kind. Jesus paid the price.

> Who hath delivered us from the power of darkness, and hath translated us into the kingdom of his dear Son.
> - Colossians 1:13 KJV

The idea of generational curses comes from God warning against idolatry.

> Thou shalt not bow down thyself to them, nor serve them: for I the LORD thy God am a jealous God, visiting the iniquity of the fathers upon the children unto the **third and fourth generation** of them that hate me
> - Exodus 20:5 KJV

But verse 6 goes on to say, "And shewing mercy unto thousands of them (generations) that love me, and keep my commandments." So, do you hate God? If not, then you have nothing to worry about. Even in the Old Covenant, He poured mercy onto those who loved Him, and did not curse them.

Other Old Testament scriptures address this, too, so it is obvious that it was of significant importance. Even though God was *slow to anger*, there were limits to His patience (Numbers 14:18). Idolatry crossed the line (Deuteronomy 5:9). But Ezekiel and Jeremiah, both prophets, foretold the day when no children would suffer for the fathers' iniquities.

> In those days, it will never again be said, 'The fathers have eaten sour grapes, and the children's teeth are set on edge.' Rather, each will die for his own iniquity. Anyone who eats sour grapes — his own teeth will be set on edge. "Look, the days are coming" — this is the Lord's declaration — "when I will make a new covenant with the house of Israel and with the house of Judah. - Jeremiah 31:29-31 CSB

Those days refers to the coming Messiah — New Covenant days. Our days. Jesus, on the cross, dealt the final blow to curses of all kinds.

> When Jesus had received the sour wine, He said, It is finished! And He bowed his head and gave up His spirit.
> - John 19:30 AMPC

That sour wine, or vinegar, broke the curse that was described as the children's teeth being set on edge to the third and fourth generation. Note that the sponge soaked in sour wine was raised up to Jesus on a branch of hyssop. Hyssop represents purification and the transfer of sins to the sacrifice. It was used to sprinkle blood on the doorposts of the Israelites' homes the night of the first Passover to protect the firstborn from the Angel of Death. This was not the only thing Jesus did at the cross that didn't involve bloodshed — He was humiliated by men and forsaken by His Father. He was stripped of his fine clothes and made poor. But taking the sour wine was His last act. You have been bought and paid for if you're a Christian. The enemy has no power over your life.

In fact, even before Jesus went to the cross, He was demonstrating the New Covenant. He knew the price He was going to pay. He was forgiving sins and healing before the cross, so you might say He was doing all this on *credit*. In John 9, Jesus encountered a man that was *blind from birth*, who we discussed earlier, and the disciples asked who had sinned to make the man be born blind — his parents or himself. Jesus told them neither had sinned. Well, they were all human, so there had to have been sin in their lives, but the point was that neither sin nor his parents had anything to do with this man's birth defect. It was just another work of the enemy. So do not be concerned about what your ancestors did — Jesus paid for their sins, too. It did not cause your disease.

What to do Under the New Covenant

We see complex trauma from childhood turning people into addicts. My dear childhood friend died at 40, the same as his dad. How can these things happen if there are no generational curses? The answer is lack of knowledge of God. You have to know that you are thoroughly cleansed and forgiven — that God has not cursed you. You have to know your authority — cast out any demon that plagues your family, and speak to any problem that seems to cling to you and your relatives, whether it be a heart condition, cancer, anger, anemia, or poverty. You have to determine in yourself that with the Holy Spirit's help, you're going to make different choices than your parents did regarding, say, abuse or addictions.

> You're a New Creation with New Blood, New DNA and a New Spirit

And know your identity! You are now a new creation, a child of The Most High God. It's His DNA (Divine Nature Attributes) in your body now, not that of your earthly ancestors. The old you is dead, crucified with Christ, and you're now part of what some translations even call a new species that had never existed before Jesus!

Bloodlines do matter, and the Blood of Jesus makes you a completely different person whether you feel it or not. You are royalty! A king and a priest, that is what God calls you.

> And hath made us kings and priests unto God and his Father; to him *be* glory and dominion for ever and ever. Amen. - Revelation 1:6 KJV

Start walking in your new identity. Nothing from the old you can touch you when you're secure in your new family.

Jesus Couldn't Heal in Nazareth

The *fact* that Jesus couldn't do miracles in His hometown has been taught and agreed with and drilled into us as long as I can remember, so no doubt it was going on for generations before. What *is* true is that familiarity breeds contempt, so no prophet is welcome in his own land, as Jesus said. My husband, who sometimes traveled the world teaching professionals in the marine industry used to tease, "You're only an expert if you're at least five hundred miles from home, and you didn't bring your wife along."

Let's take another look at Jesus' stopover in Nazareth. Matthew and Mark both give accounts of this day in Jesus' healing ministry, and the bulk of the two passages are nearly identical. But Matthew is the one we are more familiar with. Coincidentally (not), it is also the one that most gives modern readers the impression that Jesus was defeated by the people's lack of faith. Compare the two accounts:

> ...Coming to his hometown, he began teaching the people in their synagogue, and they were amazed. "Where did this man get this wisdom and these miraculous powers?" they asked. "Isn't this the carpenter's son? Isn't his mother's name Mary, and aren't his brothers James, Joseph, Simon and Judas? Aren't all his sisters with us? Where then did this man get all these things?" And they took offense at him. But Jesus said to them, "A prophet is not without honor except in his own town and in his own home." And he did not do many miracles there because of their lack of faith. - Matthew 13:53-58 NIV

> Jesus left there and went to his hometown, accompanied by his Disciples. When the Sabbath came, he began to teach in the synagogue, and many who heard him were amazed. "Where did this man get these things?" they asked. "What's this wisdom that has been given him? What are these remarkable miracles he is performing? Isn't this the carpenter? Isn't this Mary's son and the brother of James, Joseph, Judas and Simon? Aren't his sisters here with us?" And they took offense at him. Jesus said to them, "A prophet is not without honor except in his own town, among his relatives and in his own home." He could not do any miracles there, except lay his hands on a few sick people and heal them. He was amazed at their lack of faith.
> - Mark 6:1-6 NIV

Nazareth was a small town, and one most people disparaged. "Can anything good come from Nazareth?" was a popular saying of the time. You could say it was to Israel as Newfoundland is to Canada, as New Jersey is to New Yorkers, or as California is to the Deep South (and vice versa). That day, the synagogue was probably full of people who had come to hear the local boy preach.

Did you notice that early in both passages the people were exclaiming about Jesus' miracles? Then something unexpected happened. Both Matthew and Mark state, "And they took offense at Him." The outcome, as written in the Book of Matthew states, "And He did not do many miracles there because of their lack of faith." But Mark explains a little further saying, "He could not do any miracles there, except lay his hands on a few sick people and heal them." So Matthew says He didn't do many; and for some reason, people take that to mean *any*. Whereas, Mark says He laid hands on (and healed) only a few people. These details make a huge difference in how what Jesus did affects us today.

Let's say your church invites a guest speaker one Sunday morning, but before he's finished speaking, the pastor and the elders are shaking their heads in the front pews. (I have no problem imagining this scenario.) Soon, they even interrupt him mid-sentence to argue points of doctrine. They get angry, and voices are raised because this guy is contradicting their long-held beliefs and teachings in their own house! Are you going down front at the end of the service for this usurper to pray over you? No way.

He could not do any miracles there except lay his hands on a few sick people and heal them. In other words, every person He laid hands on He healed, as usual. The only problem was that there simply were not many people to lay hands on. The local rabbi and elders and most of the congregation had decided to take offense at the bastard kid of the local carpenter speaking as if He knew better than what they'd been taught all their lives. Jesus challenged a lot of long-held beliefs, so very few people allowed Jesus to minister to them that day.

We have misunderstood this event for centuries. The belief that Jesus can't make healing happen where there's a lack of faith has built up to the point of pervasiveness in the church, based on the misinterpretation of this recounting of Jesus' visit to Nazareth. It has caused untold numbers to miss out on their healing. Jesus heals everyone, every time. All you have to do is allow Him to.

Like the people of Nazareth, are some of your long-held beliefs being challenged? Lay them at Jesus' feet and let Him minister to you.

He Can Heal Some Things, but Not Your Thing

Seriously? Let me be sure I understand you. You're saying that the One Who created billions of galaxies, trillions of planets and uncountable stars, Who holds everything in place by the word of His power, Who created the human body — the intricacies of which we still cannot fathom, Who in His infinite wisdom can weave all things into good in the life of every person who loves Him, the God of angel armies, the God Who has all authority in heaven, on earth and below the earth, the God Who knows every hair on your head — HE is limited in what He can heal?

Jesus was going through all the cities and villages, teaching in their synagogues and proclaiming the gospel of the kingdom, and healing every kind of disease and every kind of sickness. - Matthew 9:35 NASB

I checked the Greek, and the word, *pas*, translated as *all* and as *every* in this scripture means… (drumroll, please) … ALL — every one, no exclusions.

ALS, MS, RSD, chicken pox, cancer (every kind), depression, heart disease, diabetes, autism, ADD/ADHD, Down's Syndrome, carpal tunnel syndrome, shingles, broken bones, metal plates and screws in the body (they disappear), phobias, old football injuries, appendicitis, colds, hormonal imbalance, flus, coronavirus, sprains, arthritis, death, kidney stones and gallstones, traumatic brain injuries, conjoined twins, preeclampsia, tooth decay, vision issues, burns, crush injuries, TMJ, migraines, toxic overload, nutritional deficiencies, parasitic infestations, every virus, brain fog, PCOS, cirrhosis, infertility — you cannot name anything that Jesus has not cured, because every name must bow to His Name, the Name Above All Names.

IF I ONLY HAD ENOUGH FAITH

Most of us have heard at one time or another that you could be healed if only you had enough faith. It's a belief that's been promulgated for decades in charismatic circles and the *word of faith* movement. Faith to be healed, the right kind of faith, enough faith, great faith — they're all familiar phrases. Have you ever stood in a line to be prayed for by a healing evangelist and been asked when it's finally your turn, "Brother, do you have enough faith to receive your healing today?"

I have good news. Jesus doesn't require your faith for you to be healed.

Cody is a Pomeranian. Yes, a dog. Every autumn for many years now, he has had an allergic reaction to something seasonal, and scratched himself silly. This fall, though, it was much worse than usual. He scratched constantly. He couldn't walk from one end of the house to the other without stopping several times to scratch. He scratched until he bled. His long, fine fur was matted and stuck to his skin by the blood. He had patches of bare, raw skin where there should have been fur. He couldn't sleep, such was the necessity to scratch. For three weeks this poor dog went without sleep, and nothing brought relief. Normally playful, loving, and welcoming to visitors, Cody was exhausted, moody, snappish, growling, tail down, and miserable. It was pitiful. One day, his human mom snatched him up into her lap, held him tight, and prayed a desperate prayer over him, asking the Holy Spirit to reach into her pet and heal him. Cody jumped down from her lap, and promptly went to sleep. He slept for hours. And hours. And he has not scratched since. His fur has grown back, he's alert, playful, and happy again.

Remember the two people in the Bible that Jesus said had great faith? They were Gentiles, not filtering the perceived likelihood of healing through their knowledge of the law, through whether they thought they were holy enough or deserving enough. (See "in Chapter 11, My Sins Block the Blessings.") Cody is a Gentile, in a manner of speaking. He has no knowledge of the law and no guilty conscience. But, how can it be said of a dog that he has great faith? It can't. At least not in the sense that we usually think of faith — super spiritual, something to be achieved with a lot of Bible study, prayer, seeking, beseeching, self-searching, and great effort on our part. Cody does none of that. He simply receives love. He's very good at receiving because he has confidence in his masters. He has confidence in his masters because they are good to him.

Nobody told Cody he had to have enough faith to get healed. He just received the love of The Master, Who cares for his mom — the Master Who, even in the Old Testament, promised to bless our livestock, and even watches over every sparrow.

Remember how Jesus said in Matthew 18:3 that we must come to Him as little children? Dogs and kids are quite similar in their trust. If you tell your kids to get in the car to go to Grandma's house, they don't ask if there's enough gas or if you've checked the tires. They don't ask what mood Grandma will be in when they arrive. They just jump in the car, KNOWING they'll see Grandma soon and get spoiled while there. That's how we should see our God — the overflowing Source of all good things.

Good News: You Can Get Healed Without Faith!

The first time Jesus healed on earth, that person probably didn't know Jesus from Adam's housecat. So who had the faith? Jesus did. Later, yes, people started having faith in Jesus because His reputation spread. But He started out as an unknown, just another guy from Nazareth, the same way new ministries are started today — see a need, meet it. Jesus met the needs of the sick in many ways, and the faith of the sick was only one way. Example after example in the Bible shows that only one party involved in healing needs to have faith, and it needn't be the sick person.

- Naaman, commander of the army of Syria was a leper, was told to dip himself in the Jordan seven times. He rebelled at the idea, having no faith. Then his servant basically said, "What do you have to lose?" So he dipped seven times in the Jordan and was miraculously healed.
- When four friends lowered their buddy through the ceiling on a pallet to get him before Jesus, it was the four friends' faith that Jesus commended. Scripture says nothing about whether or not the lame man had faith. As far as we know, he was just along for the ride, literally.

- Martha and Mary had no faith that their brother Lazarus would be raised from the dead — they both made that perfectly clear. They believed Jesus would have healed him if He'd arrived in time, but once Lazarus was dead, in Martha and Mary's minds, it was over. (Could that be why Jesus wept?) And how could Lazarus have had faith? He was dead.
- When the lame man sat outside the temple gate, he asked for money, not healing. But Peter and John told him to get up and walk, in Jesus' name, and he was immediately healed.

Did Jesus ever ask anyone if they had enough faith to be healed? He declared people healed. He delivered them from a spirit of infirmity and then declared them healed. He spoke freedom; He spoke life. He gave them a simple task and said they'd be healed when they followed His directions. He spoke healing from a distance. He applied mud. Some people drew healing out of Him by faith. Each is just one way to be healed. Jesus pointed out faith, but He never required faith from the sick as a prerequisite for healing.

This revelation is diametrically opposed to what many of us have always heard. You can be healed without one iota of faith. What you cannot do without faith is pray for unbelievers and see them healed. So the next time somebody asks you if you have enough faith to be healed when they're about to pray for you, tell them that's their job. The pray-er is supposed to be praying the *prayer of faith*. James 5: 14-15 confirms that. HOWEVER, if you have faith that when that person prays for you, you will be healed, then you will be, whether they actually have faith or not. The point is, only one person needs to be standing in faith.

What I am NOT saying:
- I am not saying we don't need faith.
- I am not saying faith is unnecessary in your Christian walk.
- I am not saying your faith is not a means of being healed.
- I am not saying that your faith or lack of it doesn't affect your health.

I'm only saying that your own faith is not the ONLY way to receive healing. Faith is not required of you, but it IS required of somebody.

Why did Jesus mention the great faith of the centurion and the Canaanite woman, and the faith of the woman with the issue of blood, if it's not important? It IS important. By faith you can absolutely be healed right now where you sit reading this book.

You see, Jesus could have sought that Hebrew woman out, saying, "The Father told me there is a woman in this house that has been going to doctors for twelve years trying to be healed, spending all she had and is only the worse for it. I've come to meet her need." He could have gone with the centurion to where the man's servant lay and healed him; same for the demon-possessed daughter of the Gentile woman. We need to know about faith being a vehicle to health and healing, because here we are, in the twenty-first century, with very few people having fully renewed their minds around the laying on of hands, the casting out of spirits of infirmity, and the quickening of our mortal bodies by the Holy Spirit. We need to know that we can just receive by faith. So Jesus drew our attention to our own faith as one of the ways to be healed.

Yet the wily devil has convinced the church that we have to have ENOUGH faith, as if a certain amount of faith will force God to part with some of His healing power. Wrong! Believing this, we eventually turn faith into a work instead of the confident trust it's supposed to be.

You cannot force God to do anything, so thank goodness you don't have to. God's healing power was activated in the earth over two thousand years ago because He loved all the people of His creation so very much.

Faith is a magnet that attracts grace, just as fear attracts calamity. It pleases God when you get healed, and it's impossible to achieve that without faith — your's or another's.

Have Confidence in Jesus He Has Enough Faith for All of Us

How can we have been so wrong about this burdensome faith prerequisite for so long? It's the same as so many other doctrines the scriptures prove wrong. Man fails in his own strength and self-effort, then makes up an excuse for failure based loosely on scriptures taken out of context. And every time man does that, he puts more responsibility for the outcome on man, so that man's responsibility in receiving grace becomes bigger and bigger and God's part becomes smaller and smaller in our eyes. Therefore, we succeed less and less in receiving God's grace, and the devil just stands back and laughs at our inability to utilize what God has already given us.

I have two tips for you if you're feeling you don't have enough faith to receive, or have made standing in faith into a work of the flesh in trying to get ENOUGH faith to see results:

Pray in tongues. Scripture tells us that allowing the Spirit to intercede for you prays perfect prayers, imparts wisdom, knowledge, and revelation, builds your faith, and edifies your body — all of which will help you be healed and stay healed.

Faith is trust and confidence in God. Just change the word! Just say you have confidence in Jesus. You'll find that the use of a different word provides the freedom to rest in His finished work. Now THAT'S FAITH!

Give up trying to have *enough faith* — just know that Jesus has more than enough to cover you, that His blood has already paid for your healing, and that the Father loves you beyond measure. Then without realizing it, you have faith! It's unconscious faith. It's confidence in Jesus. Call it confidence and suddenly you have it, without having to work for it at all.

CHAPTER 15
Praying ". . .if It Be Thy Will"

This is a hot button for me. I cringe every time I hear someone pray, "Heal him, Father, if it be Thy will." That prayer is not only ineffective, it's damaging — ineffective because there's no faith for a good outcome behind it, and damaging because both the prayer and its inevitable outcome undermine the faith of everyone within hearing. If you don't know His will on any given subject, you simply cannot have faith for it. So please, just don't pray until you can pray in faith. You are praying double-minded prayers and will not be able to receive anything from God.

> But he must ask in faith, without doubting, because he who doubts is like a wave of the sea, blown and tossed by the wind. That man should not expect to receive anything from the Lord. - James 1:6,7 BSB

Have you ever thought when reading this familiar passage that it seemed just a tiny bit mean-spirited of God? Look again. It does not say that God is withholding, only that we're not receiving.

Millions of Christians around the world believe that there are times that healing is just not part of God's plan. Sometimes He heals; sometimes He doesn't. Then when the person dies (no surprise there), we make excuses for God's *calling him home.* We say things like, "God wanted that beautiful little child for His garden in heaven," and "He was such a good man, God must have needed him up there." Hopefully though, having gotten this far in the book, it is settled in your soul what God's will is — that we all live and "proclaim the works of the Lord" (Psalm 118:17).

If it be thy will... is obviously calling His will for the sick person into question — a question fully and repeatedly answered in the scriptures. You know better now. God has proven over and over through His Word that He WANTS you healed and that, in fact, your healing was accomplished at the cross more than two thousand years ago.

I'm repeating myself, I know — but this is vitally important: God is infinite. He has infinite ways to accomplish His will in the earth through us. He has no need for those plans to include sickbeds for a single one of His children. How can I say that? I'm not saying it. God said it, over and over in the Word. He created us the way He wanted us — as eternal physical beings living in peace and joy, communing with Him without any disease or sin surrounded by beauty and every provision we could ever dream of. That is what He created, so that is His will. And then we messed it up — so Jesus came, dealt with sin, and healed us all.

You must KNOW it is God's will that you be whole. Until you settle the issue of God's will around healing, you may as well stop praying about it, because you cannot pray a prayer of faith. However, you can certainly pray for His help in understanding His will and acting on it. Remember Jesus' instructions — pray that the Father's will as it is demonstrated in heaven be done on earth.

Creation Reveals God's Will for Man, and God's Will Never Changes

Everything I'm sharing with you in this book is backed up by scripture. More precisely, scripture is dictating what I share with you in this book, scripture that the Holy Spirit has been opening up to me every hour I spend researching. If you still believe God doesn't always want to heal His children, and you want to keep believing that and promulgating it, then you need to find the scriptures to support it. They're not there. There is no New Covenant basis for that belief, quite simply because Jesus provided healing for everyone when he took the scourging.

Where the will of God has been made clear in the scriptures, you must eliminate the practice of insulting Him by praying, "...if it be Thy will." He's already told you what His will is, and He has told you to get busy enforcing that perfect will in your life and in the whole earth.

Part Five
Your Transformed Mind in Action

...for this reason, we must pay attention all the more to what we have heard, so that we will not drift away.
- Hebrews 2:1 CSB

Give me life in accordance with your faithful love, and I will obey the decrees you have spoken. Lord, your word is forever; it is firmly fixed in heaven. Your faithfulness is for all generations...If your instruction had not been my delight, I would have died in my affliction.
- Psalm 119:88-92 CSB

...their fear and reverence for Me are a commandment of men that is learned by repetition [without any thought as to the meaning]. Therefore, behold! **I will again do marvelous things with this people**, marvelous and astonishing things; and the wisdom of their wise men will perish, and the understanding of their discerning men will vanish *or* be hidden. - Isaiah 29:13 AMPC

CHAPTER 16
Hope Again

Can anyone still have an errant lingering notion that God might use illness to chastise you, teach you a lesson, somehow get glory for Himself, or to achieve some other unknown mysterious end game we can't understand because His ways and thoughts are higher than ours? I just don't think it's possible.

Being rid of wrong beliefs brings new levels of freedom, and it is for freedom that Jesus set us free (Romans 5:1). You can see the truth because the Holy Spirit is causing the scales to fall away from your eyes. Burdens drop off of you, and you can breathe easier, finally beginning to recognize that ONLY good comes from your heavenly Father.

Now add to that this knowledge: When you accepted Jesus, God put Himself into you — right down into your very spirit. Then He put You into Jesus. So now, when He looks at you, He doesn't see what's wrong with you, He sees His perfect Son, whom you are becoming more and more like. He can see what's missing in you — the blanks He wants to fill in for you. But He doesn't see them as problems or sins because God is not sin or problem-oriented. He's promise, provision, and possibility-oriented. All your shortcomings, flaws, and the obstacles you need solutions for, including illness, are simply places where you're missing something — revelation, understanding, a sense of vision or purpose, provision you haven't received. Don't worry about what you do wrong or problems that life is throwing at you, just think about the promises, provision, and possibilities that God has already put in place for you. His provision says you can reign over the problem and even profit from it. Don't focus on the problem. Focus on God and what He has for you in each circumstance. Remember that what you think about most is what you begin to have faith in. What you gaze at, you begin to look like. So keep your eyes on Jesus. You can allow your illness to grow in your mind to the point that it appears insurmountable. Or you can know that your God Who loves you, Who melts mountains and forms suns with His words, has provided you with perfect health and a specific purpose for the long life you were created for.

> "It is Written" and "In Jesus' Name" Are the Most Powerful Words on Earth

It's time to change some habits. Make it your mission going forward to speak only what God says over any given situation. Speak God's Word as Jesus did in the wilderness. Agree with Him. You will begin to think His thoughts — you have the mind of Christ, after all. The Holy Spirit will help.

The devil can only steal what you already have. Disease isn't so much you being made sick, but the health Jesus already gave you being stolen — **attempted** theft. He knows Jesus healed you before he even tried to make you sick! It's all deception. But God makes His kids MORE than just conquerors — He won the war for us, and we get to walk among the enemies, collecting the spoils, while they stand helplessly chained, watching what they stole from us being taken back with interest. How do you get to that point?

This book is not meant to be a "how to receive healing" book, though many will be healed instantly by the removal of wrong beliefs. However, I can't just leave you hanging when it comes to practical application of truths the scriptures have revealed to you. Here are some of our weapons of spiritual warfare:

Go on the Offensive

1. Instead of crying to God about your problem, tell the problem about your God. We deceive ourselves when we wait for God's promises to drop into our laps instead of DOING what the Word says — take authority, exercise your dominion.

2. Speak aloud and tell the devil you are the Redeemed and he has no authority in your life, that he's a squatter and you're evicting him. Quote the Word to him. Fight the devil with the Word of God — the sword of the spirit. Tell him, "It is written…" the same way Jesus did in the wilderness. If you don't know much scripture yet, start with, "By His stripes I am healed" and then learn more. Have comebacks ready for every lie he whispers in your ear, no matter who's mouth it comes through. Be sure to speak TO the mountain, too — the pain, the tumor, the blood sugar level, the blurry vision. Jesus said,

Faith It 'til You Make It

> "Truly I tell you that if anyone SAYS to this mountain…and has NO DOUBT in his heart but BELIEVES that it will happen, it will be done for him." - Mark 11:23 BSB

3. If you don't fully believe the truth yet, say it even more! You can speak yourself into believing a lot faster than you can believe yourself into speaking. Your words are your artillery. This is of prime importance because your words are your most effective weapon when mixed with faith. Preach to yourself while you tell the devil where to go.

4. Scripture tells us "angels hearken to the voice of His Word" (Psalm 103:20). That means that when you speak (give voice to) the scriptures, angels set about doing His will that you just spoke. The same can be said about dark angels when you speak God's word in authority against their works. They have to obey it.

> Authority: Jesus Has It ALL. The Enemy Has None — Zero, Zip, Nada. So Fear Not.

5. Don't forget your medicine — the Word of God. Set your alarm as you would to take prescribed drugs on schedule, and read those healing scriptures aloud. Confess them over your body. You have authority over your body. Write them on index cards and tape them on your bathroom mirror, your refrigerator, and your dashboard. Keep them in front of your eyes. Now mix them with faith!

> "...but the word which they heard did not profit them, not being mixed with faith…" - Hebrews 4:2 NKJV

6. Praise Him! Praise Him for Who He is, for the great things He has done, and for the outcome you know is being accomplished right now. Praising Him builds up your faith and routs out the devil — he'll take off with his tail between his legs.

Defensive Measures

7. Be watchful over your words. Stop saying things like, "My feet are killing me," and "That cheesecake is to die for." No, I'm not joking. We are created in God's image, and so our words are creative like His. We don't have perfect faith, so they don't work as quickly, that's all. Remember: "Death and life are in the power of the tongue, and those who love it and

indulge it will eat its fruit and bear the consequences of their words" (Proverbs 18:21 AMP). Don't curse yourself!

8. Deal with negative thoughts as soon as they pop up, so that those seeds cannot take root, grow, and become destructive — they're like kudzu. (If you're not from the Deep South, look it up.) Put on the helmet of salvation to protect your thought life. When you have an unproductive thought, picture yourself grabbing it mid-air and throwing it at Jesus' feet. He will stomp it and use it as a footstool. Trust me; this really works. God said He was tickled pink when I started doing this, and that it was making a notable difference.

> ### Your Healing is More Real in the Spirit Realm Than Your Illness is in the Physical

9. Stay spiritually minded, focusing on what is true in the spirit realm — what the Word reveals. In the spiritual realm, you are whole. Being ruled by your five senses is being carnally minded. You must believe the Word of God more than you believe the doctors, more than you believe the symptoms, sometimes more than you believe your spouse or pastor.

> "For the mind set on the flesh is death, but the mind set on the Spirit is life and peace" - Romans 8:6 NASB

> ### Passivity is Permission for the Enemy to Make Himself at Home

10. The enemy cannot hurt you without your cooperation. You have to agree with him and his lying symptoms, to be sick. The devil takes your passivity as permission. So tell him you choose not to participate in his scheme. Tell him, "NO!"

Tactical Maneuvers

11. Learn more about your identity in Christ — who you really are and what you really have. It always helps our minds to receive when you understand WHY God has given you already what you're seeking. And it'll do wonders for our outlook on life — better than DECADES of therapy.

12. Jesus has signed His power of attorney over to you. That's your authority. Everything you speak in His Name that is within the will of the Father MUST come to pass, because it is effectively Jesus speaking. Wow, but true. If you have to speak it multiple times, so be it. But speak it in faith, expecting the intended result. The process will move faster as you learn to speak only truth in your everyday life – no exaggerations, and no idle curses. Your words are just as important to God as Jesus' are, and there are many scriptures showing how important it is to God to back up the words of those who love Him.

13. Authority and faith are the power twins. This book is not big enough to delve deeper into these subjects. For now, just remember that faith is not about you working, it's about you resting.

14. Even though it may sound contradictory, James 2:26 says, "Faith without works is dead!" Blind Bartimaeus threw off the cloak that branded him a beggar and moved toward Jesus' voice. That is the type of *work* that *faith without works* refers to. That action — like my husband wearing a type of shoe he couldn't wear before his leg grew out — demonstrates your faith and sucks healing out of the spirit realm and into the now.

15. Get baptized in the Holy Spirit and pray in tongues. Praying in tongues edifies you—builds you up physically as well as in your soul (1 Corinthians 14:4), keeps you centered in God's love, and builds up your most holy faith (Jude 1:20 CSB). And it's free. What a deal!

16. Take communion. I will address this subject from different perspectives and in more detail in a subsequent books, but for now, think about this: there was never a more vibrant and healthy man on this earth than Jesus. He gave that body to be scourged for our healing. He is called the Bread of Life, and the Children's Bread is healing and deliverance. He instructed, "Do this in remembrance of Me." But He's never told us to do anything for Him that didn't also provide benefits for us. Communion is not a ritual to be performed; it is a blessing to be received. "Take, eat."

17. Read my next book.

18. Love Jesus and spend time letting Him love on you. Nothing is more life-affirming.

The whole question of God's will toward healing is answered in this one red-letter passage:

> The thief comes only in order to steal and kill and destroy. I came that they may have and ENJOY life, and have it in abundance (to the full, till it overflows).
> - John 10:10 AMP

Those words are your measuring stick going forward. Whatever circumstance or question or thought you're staring at, ask yourself this, *does it bring life?* If it doesn't, then it's either from your carnal mind, or it's from the enemy, but it is not from God. So wage war on it. Never give up, never surrender (Galatians 6:9).

Can you absorb one more truth before I share the open vision God gave me? Here goes... Jesus gave us dominion over all the works of the enemy, not over people. That's a proof of this truth: it's not really about you, after all. If healing was about specific people, we would have a list of questions to ask before ministering healing. We don't have authority over any person. We only have authority over 1) evil spirits and 2) evil works. No matter who you are, no matter what you've done, no matter what disease or condition you're facing, **your health challenge is a work of the enemy and God wants it destroyed**. Yes, He loves you and doesn't want you to suffer, but He wants to kill that disease no matter who has it. If there was a case of ragweed allergy standing in the middle of the road, not bothering anyone, Jesus would tell you to squash it like a bug. Jesus said He came to destroy the works of the devil. Let Him.

CHAPTER 17
The Vision

Here's the thing: the closer we get to Jesus' return, the more revelation God unlocks for us. So when you hear something you've never heard before, don't just assume it's from the devil. Goodness knows we've been attributing the devil's work to God for generations (*acts of God*, taking loved ones for *His garden in heaven*, etc.). Take new perspectives to the Lord, and ask Him.

What I am about to share, well, some of it is just plain off the chart. You'll probably think some of it sounds completely outrageous — I felt the same way as I was receiving it.

> That's the Way It Often Is with God — You Hear, You Do, and THEN You Understand

Some of it I should have known already (see Chapter 11, I'm Not Worthy). I thought I knew it but hadn't applied it yet; so I didn't really understand it. Some of the principles you've already read in the pages of this book. Other parts of the vision are so radical that months after the fact, I still haven't wrapped my brain around them. I'm still renewing *my* mind, just like you. So it's only for the sake of obedience that I step out on that limb and share this now, at His instruction. Please don't burn me at the stake.

The pain was so intense I found myself wishing to be in labor, or having a gallbladder attack, instead. Every time I was prayed over by others it got worse, which just confirmed to me that it was a spiritual attack. So I counterattacked, but the pain and lack of sleep had worn me down. Is anything worse than an abscessed tooth? Because I was writing this book, I dug my heels in even deeper and stubbornly refused to go to the dentist. *It's just You and me, God.* I gave in on my anti-pain medication stance pretty quickly, but it didn't help a bit. Codeine (over-the-counter in Canada), clove oil, Oragel, nothing touched it.

Lord, I know it's not Your will that I be in pain. It's not Your will that I lack health in any way. This pain is here illegally. I rebuke the enemy and his plans against me. He's trying to convince me that I have no right to publish this book, but he's a liar. I know my calling, and the enemy cannot discourage me. I speak to this pain and tell it to GO NOW in the mighty Name of Jesus. And on it went for days. There were periods of relief. One was when my friend sat in my living room praying in tongues for five hours while I finally slept. But the pain returned.

Meanwhile, between naps and bouts of pacing the floor in agony, I'd been pondering two subjects, asking the Lord for clarity.

1. I'd heard a pastor I admire state that God is pouring His grace out on the entire world, 24/7. My immediate reaction, I'm ashamed to say, was, *Don't you mean on the Christians?* I had an elitist mindset I hadn't even been aware of.

2. A friend told me of a post she'd seen on Pinterest. A non-believer wrote that she'd been healed of systemic candida overgrowth simply by deciding she didn't have it. She'd been going to the doctor regularly, adhering to the ever-so-strict candida diet and doing everything the doctor told her to do for many months with no improvement. She was finally fed up. The post said her reaction was: "I'm done. I do NOT have candida." She stormed out of the doctor's office and went straight to a bar and ordered a margarita — pretty much the worst thing you can do when fighting candida.

Huh. She decided to believe she didn't have it, and she stuck to that belief as strongly as she had to the candida regimen the months before. She went back to her normal lifestyle and her normal diet. Her only change was in her mindset. She returned to her doctor for the next scheduled appointment, and he could find no trace of candida overgrowth.

On the eighth day, I was so used to the pain it had lost its hold on me. *Lord, I know that when I come out of this, and I will because of Your great love for me, You will have shown me something — something of great importance, something fresh, something that's just for this book. You'll show me what I'm missing.*

Ninth day: *Lord I don't even care about the pain anymore. It hasn't killed me. I just want to know what you have for the book.*

On the tenth morning of the toothache, I woke suddenly, sat up, and heard two bell tones in my head. *Ding. Ding.* The answers to my questions began downloading.

1. *Of course the Lord is pouring out grace on the entire world! Duh. Nobody could get saved if He wasn't.* What had I been thinking? In the moment that I'd heard that statement from the pastor, I'd been thinking of all the blessings we receive after we accept Christ, so the statement had struck me the wrong way. I was ignoring the main reason for grace — the remission of

sin. Here's where the surprise revelation came in. This meant that all the other things that grace, the undeserved favor of God, comprises — peace, joy, love, the mind of Christ, healing, protection, prosperity, wisdom, deliverance, security, promotion, etc. — all these things were in continuous flow to EVERYONE, not just to Christians. *For God so loved THE WORLD.* Rain falls on the just and the unjust.

> The Lord is good to all, and His tender mercies are over all His works [the entirety of things created].
> - Psalm 145:9 AMP

2. Regarding unbelievers getting healed, I remembered hearing as a girl of a wealthy man who'd received one of those death-sentence diagnoses — ALS, I think. He proceeded to treat himself by watching slapstick comedy all day every day, laughing all day long. He was applying a Biblical principle: laughter doeth good like a medicine (Proverbs 17:22). I thought of a leading financial expert who taught personal money management skills to people of all socio-economic levels. I'd once heard a friend comment, "Of course it works — they're teaching Biblical financial principles, whether they realize it or not."

Do Biblical principles work no matter who applies them? Believing that you are healed works, if this lady's story is true, even when you're not giving credit to the One who provided it. This may not sound right to you — it didn't to me. Wow. That would take a lot of pressure off, wouldn't it? It would confirm that you don't have to be worthy to get healed. Then I had another not-very-Christlike thought: *If some heathen can get healed instantly, I'm dang sure not letting it pass me by!* (Another elitism, but it didn't change the fact that God wants me well.)

My thoughts began to sound not only selfish, but heretical to my churched ears: So, normally, we walk to the front of the sanctuary and accept what the church generally calls salvation — eternal life in heaven through the remission of sins — and leave the rest at the altar — healing, provision, and everything else Christ accomplished for us. We don't know any better. We're not taught that all the other things are part of salvation (sozo). That means that theoretically, we could accept only healing, or only provision, and leave forgiveness and eternal life at the altar. It would be stupid, but in theory we should be able to. Apparently, that's what the rich man and the lady with candida did. Then again, how dumb is it that we accept the most important component but don't receive all the other lesser blessings that are part of the abundant life here on earth?

I questioned the Lord. *This can't possibly be right.* But He is so much bigger and so much better than we believe.

What I was hearing went against a lot of widely accepted beliefs, including beliefs I was raised on. If it was God speaking, though, then it's true. I had specifically asked God those two questions, and I'd asked Him for something special for this book.

> "So I say to you, ask, and it will be given to you; seek, and you will find; knock, and it will be opened to you. For everyone who asks receives, and he who seeks finds, and to him who knocks it will be opened. If a son asks for bread from any father among you, will he give him a stone? Or if he asks for a fish, will he give him a serpent instead of a fish? - Luke 11: 9-10 NKJV

OK, so this is You, Lord. Then I'm listening. Boiling it down, I was hearing God say that healing is available for everyone, not just believers. Anyone.

This is hard to believe, Lord. Not that you heal unbelievers — you do that all the time through street healers and evangelists and pastors. But that's when somebody is praying over them in Jesus' Name. You're saying you can just believe for healing, and be healed? Anybody? Even when they don't even know to thank you?

All I was experiencing that morning is simply the practical application of the truths He'd been showing me in the Word, that sin and sickness are root and fruit, same for forgiveness and healing, and they're all part of one transaction. If forgiveness is available to every person ever to live, then so is healing. And He did not un-heal the lepers that failed to say, "Thank you." Jesus heals them all because it is the Father's will to destroy the works of the devil wherever they are found.

> You know of Jesus of Nazareth, how God anointed Him with the Holy Spirit and with power, and how He went about doing good and healing all who were oppressed by the devil, for God was with Him. - Acts 10:38 NASB

I should know this already. I know plenty of people who minister healing to strangers, including unbelievers. But why, Lord? Why not put a qualifier on grace that says you can only access all the lesser blessings like healing and provision if you first accept Jesus? Because it is His goodness that leads us to repentance! And because it's His nature and His desire to relieve suffering. And because the Kingdom advances with every evil work that is reversed.

Can't you see that his kindness is intended to turn you from your sin? - Romans 2:4 NLT

The Lord is good to everyone. He showers compassion on all His creation. - Psalm 145:9 NLT

But God - so rich is He in His mercy! Because of and in order to satisfy the great and wonderful and intense love with which He loved us... - Ephesians 2:4 AMPC

He is the propitiation for our sins, and not for ours only but also for the sins of the whole world. - 1 John 2:2 ESV

What Sounded Heretical to My Churched Ears Was God's Love in Action — Classic Mistake

Healing is the dinner bell to salvation — healing as evangelism — I talked about that early in the book. With the vision, God was simply showing me the culmination of things I'd already learned — the end result. He was showing me the big picture, and the playing-out of these truths, putting all the pieces together for me. Jesus saves sinners, so He heals sinners, too, by the same grace and the same transaction. Because Jesus healed unbelievers, you can lay on hands and heal an unbeliever, and an unbeliever can use his own belief that he is well to access healing and pull it into the physical realm. All this is possible because this is the way God set it up to work. He set His healing power in motion and will never recall it. No limits. *God so loved the WORLD.* What sounded heretical was God's love in action. "Come, all who are heavy laden" (Matthew 11:28). Well then, just go ahead and say it with me — "If a heathen can have it, I'm not gonna miss out!"

Then, I saw a landscape in front of me. Tan sand and stone peeked out from under green spring foliage on a sweeping plain, and a line of distant low mountains pointed to the cloudless blue. It was like a postcard that filled my vision, yet I was starting the shower running, making an attempt at brushing my abscessed tooth, etc. *Is that Israel, Lord?* Then the cross appeared, hanging over the plain, drawn in black Sharpie. *Yep, Israel.* It just hung in the air, and then it had short black lines around it depicting light, or more precisely, grace, radiating from it. The phrase 'waves of grace' came to mind. *You know, they don't really look like waves, Lord.* And so He changed my perspective. He'd certainly done that intellectually that morning already, but this time He changed it in a literal, visual way. The cross turned so that I saw it from an angle instead of straight on, and my mouth dropped open.

The rays of grace were now revealed completely, and they ARE waves. They undulate, like sine waves on the screen of an oscilloscope, up and down in perfect rolling rhythm. Understanding came. *They've been flowing out from the cross like this for over two thousand years! They're all around me, maybe even passing right through me.* I held out my hand, wondering if I could feel them flowing between my fingers, or if I would see them pass through my palm. I was in awe. *The atmosphere must be completely saturated after two thousand years of this. The earth really IS filled with His glory! The whole atmosphere is full of healing and every blessing. I could just breathe healing in!*

I took a deep breath. Instantly, all the pain and swelling in my face and jaw ran down my side to the floor, forming an invisible puddle.

God's grace exploded over the earth like a massive, eternal chain reaction when Jesus rose from the dead. It engulfed our entire world, saturating our atmosphere, clinging to each and every person hoping to be allowed in.

Take a deep breath.

...The man took Jesus at His word and departed.
- John 4:50 NIV

Acknowledgements

I'm a writer. Yet I cannot find the words to describe the magnitude of my volunteer editor's kind heart, of the work she put into this book, which far exceeded what either of us expected it to entail, nor of the gratitude that I feel toward her. Jan Youmans Mason is the wife of my dad's first cousin. Some would say that makes her a distant relative, but there is nothing distant about her. Jan is one of those rare people who manifests the gift of Helps and the heart of a servant. She is one of my favorite people in the world, and this is not the first time she's come to my rescue. There's a rather long and miraculous story of how she became my editor, and it was all God. You read a testimony of Jan's experience after hearing just a fraction of what this to-be-edited book contains, so God, as He does, blessed us both with this brilliant plan. I hope you recognize that this project is her ministry to you. Jan, thank you.

There are many others I want to recognize and thank. My mom, Charlotte Scherer Battles, has been a constant encouragement, even though my telephone rants and preaching have no doubt pushed her far outside her denominational comfort zone. Still, she has hung in there. Thanks, Mom.

Our friends Elgin and Cheryl McKillop were the first ones to read the draft of the book, and their enthusiasm was such a blessing and encouragement.

Since the writing was completed, family, friends and ministers have read and approved the final draft, and their approval gave me the determination to push for the finish line, through the ordeal of publishing and marketing. To all of those I say, the blessing that this book will be to so many will be due in part to you. Thank you all.

Bible Translations and Copyrights

It is the glory of God to conceal a thing: but the honour of kings *is* to search out a matter. - Proverbs 25:2 KJV

AMP and AMPC - Amplified Bible and Amplified Bible Classic Edition
Scripture quotations taken from the Amplified® Bible (AMP), Copyright © 2015 by The Lockman Foundation, Scripture quotations taken from the Amplified® Bible (AMPC), Copyright © 1954, 1958, 1962, 1964, 1965, 1987 by The Lockman Foundation. Both used by permission.

ASV - American Standard Version (public domain)

BSB - Berean Study Bible
The Holy Bible, Berean Study Bible, BSB
Copyright ©2016, 2018 by Bible Hub
Used by Permission. All Rights Reserved Worldwide.

CJB - Complete Jewish Bible
By David H. Stern. Copyright © 1998. All rights reserved. Used by permission of Messianic Jewish Publishers, 6120 Day Long Lane, Clarksville, MD 21029. www.messianicjewish.net.

CSB - Christian Standard Bible
Scripture quotations marked CSB have been taken from the Christian Standard Bible®, Copyright © 2017 by Holman Bible Publishers. Used by permission. Christian Standard Bible•, and CSB® are federally registered trademarks of Holman Bible Publishers

ESV - English Standard Version
Scripture quotations marked ESV are from the ESV® Bible (The Holy Bible, English Standard Version®), copyright© 2001 by Crossway Bibles, a publishing ministry of Good News Publishers. Used by permission. All rights reserved.

GNT - The Good News Translation
Scripture quotations marked (GNT) are from the Good News Translation in Today's English Version- Second Edition Copyright © 1992 by American Bible Society. Used by Permission.

GW - God's Word Translation
GOD'S WORD is a copyrighted work of God's Word to the Nations. Quotations are used by permission. Copyright© 1995 by God's Word to the Nations. All rights reserved.

KJV - King James Version (public domain)

MEV - Modern English Version
Scripture taken from the Modern English Version. Copyright © 2014 by Military Bible Association. Used by permission. All rights reserved.

NASB - New American Standard Bible
Scripture quotations taken from the New American Standard Bible (NASB), Copyright © 1960, 1962, 1963, 1968, 1971, 1972, 1973, 1975, 1977, 1995 by The Lockman Foundation
Used by permission. www.Lockman.org

NHEB - New Heart English Bible (public domain)

NIV - New International Version
THE HOLY BIBLE, NEW INTERNATIONAL VERSION®, NIV® Copyright © 1973, 1978, 1984, 2011 by Biblica, Inc.™ Used by permission. All rights reserved worldwide.

NLT - New Living Translation
Holy Bible, New Living Translation, copyright © 1996, 2004, 2015 by Tyndale House Foundation. Used by permission of Tyndale House Publishers, Inc., Carol Stream, Illinois 60188. All rights reserved.

NKJV - New King James Version
Scripture taken from the New King James Version®. Copyright © 1982 by Thomas Nelson. Used by permission. All rights reserved.

WET - Wuest Expanded Translation of the New Testament. Copyright © 1961 William B Eerdmans Publishing Co. All Rights reserved. Used with permission.

YLT - Young's Literal Translation (public domain)

www.ingramcontent.com/pod-product-compliance
Lightning Source LLC
Chambersburg PA
CBHW072155100526
44589CB00015B/2233